LIFE LINE

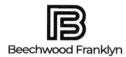

Beechwood Franklyn

Published in the UK in 2021 by Beechwood Franklyn
Copyright © Dr. Barry Monk 2021

Paperback   ISBN 978-1-8384949-0-2
eBook   ISBN 978-1-8384949-1-9

Cover design and typeset by SpiffingCovers.com

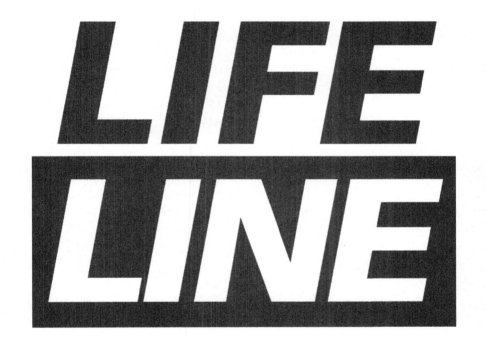

Dr Barry Monk

Foreword by Professor Harold Ellis

FOREWORD

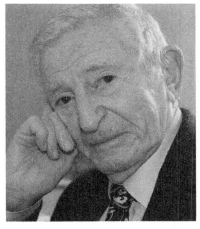

It was my great pleasure to be invited by Dr Barry Monk to write the Foreword to his fascinating book. I have to declare an interest in that I am Barry's uncle and that I was Professor of Surgery at the old Westminster Medical School in Horseferry Road, now a block of luxury apartments, when Barry arrived there as a medical student all those years ago.

'Lifeline' is made up of a series of essays on our health service on the broadest sense. The NHS began as a remarkable experiment in the concept of universal healthcare, being forced through a reluctant medical profession in July 1948 by a remarkable young man, Aneurin Bevan, the Minister of Health. Bevan famously said 'I stuffed their mouths with gold' in reference to the generous financial terms he offered to the hospital consultants and to the senior general practitioners.

It so happened that this was the very month that I qualified in Medicine and commenced my own career in surgery at the old Radcliffe Infirmary in Oxford.

The chapters cover a wide range of topics. Thus air crashes and nuclear disasters, and their forensic investigation, may throw light on human medical accidents and their causes. The vast majority of doctors in this country are hardworking and competent, but Barry investigates, with clinical precision, the stories of fake and devious doctors and their trials. Most NHS administrators are dedicated and effective, but Barry recounts some dreadful cases that have occurred where 'keeping within the budget' has resulted in hospital disasters or where junior doctors have been made to bear the burden of blame for medical catastrophes.

Finally, Barry bemoans the demise of postmortem examinations in hospitals and, with it, the loss of an invaluable tool of medical education. I hope that you will enjoy reading and learning from this book as much as I have done.

Harold Ellis, CBE, FRCS

Emeritus Professor of Surgery, University of London

December 2020

ACKNOWLEDGEMENTS

This book would never have seen the light of day but for the skilled and patient team at Spiffing Covers who turned a raw manuscript into the final product. They have shown wonderful professionalism at every stage in the process, and remarkable forbearance when I have been floundering.

I am most grateful to my uncle, Professor Harold Ellis, for providing the foreword, and also for his help and encouragement throughout the writing process. Harold has been a wonderful mentor to me over the years, just as he has to countless medical students and junior doctors.

It was Phil Coleman (see Chapter 4), master of the traditional art of print journalism, who first sowed the seeds of the idea of my writing a book about the NHS. My friend, Jill Stephen, patiently explained the principles of English spelling, grammar and punctuation that I appear to have missed out on at school.

I have been fortunate to have worked, over the years, with some wonderful colleagues, and I am grateful for their kindness and support. Many of them have helped me with background information. I will not mention individual names, because some, especially those who were directly involved in a number of the events that I have described, have asked me to respect their confidentiality.

The NHS, for all its problems, is a wonderful organisation, and I am proud to have played a small part in it. It is still a privilege to be able to help people, and I am most grateful to my present team of Hazel, Hilary and Linsay who somehow manage to keep me out of mischief (not always an easy task), and who continue to make work such a pleasure.

Nearer to home, I must thank David, Ally and Anna who constantly reassure me about my lack of computer skills and always manage to put things in perspective. I must also mention my late brother Mark, still much missed, who had a lifelong love of books and of learning and who taught me so much about medicine from the patient's perspective.

Last, but of course, not least, is Margaret, who has had a quite special place in my life, and who makes it all worthwhile.

Barry Monk

February 2021

CHAPTER 1

The NHS and Me

This book is about the NHS, but in a sense, it is also about me. In 1969, as a 17-year-old on my gap year, I spent several months working as a hospital laboratory assistant before going off to study medicine. I finally retired from the NHS in January 2020, after 33 years as a consultant dermatologist. I had worked for the NHS in the 1960s, 70s, 80s, 90s, 2000s, 2010s and 2020s. I am not sure that many of those who follow me will be able to match that. It has been an immense privilege, and along the way I have had some remarkable colleagues and wonderful patients. I am proud of what the NHS has achieved, and for my own modest part in it. But as I look back, I sometimes worry about the NHS of the future, and I do not think that I am alone in having these concerns.

My school days are now something of a distant memory. Education has changed and I am not sure how any of my teachers would have coped with modern political correctness. We were taught Latin by a fearsome man called the Reverend 'Boggy' Marsh, who wreaked terrifyingly violent punishments on anyone who made any mistakes in translations. We thought that it was slightly strange that Mr Cornish taught us German by getting us to sing Second World War German Army marching songs, especially as half the class was Jewish. It is only recently that I discovered that, in fact, he had been a war hero. He ended up a prisoner of war in Colditz Castle, but was not permitted to be one of the ill-fated escapees, as it was thought it would be safer if there were a fluent German speaker among those who stayed behind. After the war he served with the War Crimes Interrogation Unit, and was later assigned to be the liaison officer for Field Marshall Albert Kesselring at his trial. By contrast, dealing with a bunch of bumptious schoolboys must have seemed like a walk in the park.

Horace Brearley taught maths. His career as a cricketer had been cut short by the War.[1] In 1941, stationed in South Africa, he was supposed to have embarked on HMS *Hood* but was delayed and missed its departure. Not long afterwards, a German battleship sank *Hood* with only three survivors of the 1,400 people on board. Again, we knew nothing of this at the time, but he encouraged us to always be grateful for the opportunities that came our way.

I started thinking of studying medicine when I was about 14, inspired by a popular TV drama series, *Dr Finlay's Casebook*, the early scripts of which were written by the doctor and writer, AJ Cronin. Cronin's 1937 novel, *The Citadel*, which exposed the inequalities of medical care at the time, had sparked controversy in its day. There were calls for him to be thrown out of the medical profession but, nevertheless, it is said that the book had inspired Aneurin Bevan in his creation of the NHS (National Health Service).

---

1   He played one match for Yorkshire, batting with Len Hutton in 1937, and twice more, for Middlesex, in 1948.

Dr Finlay was portrayed as an enthusiastic young GP working in a rather idyllic part of rural Scotland and trying to instil some modern medical ideas into his senior colleague, the rather gruff Dr Cameron. I think the thing that really clinched the idea of a career in medicine was that, every morning before they set out on their rounds, Finlay in a splendid *Bullnose* Morris, they both tucked into a full cooked breakfast, served up by their devoted housekeeper, Janet. Today's junior doctors will be astonished to find that when I did my first job as a house surgeon at Westminster Hospital in 1975, we were indeed served a cooked breakfast in the junior doctors' mess. We needed it because it would usually be a long time before we had a chance to get anything else to eat. If you were on duty at night you were entitled to go down to the kitchens at midnight to get a hot meal, usually a decidedly unhealthy fry up, a luxury that has long disappeared.

Having decided that I wanted to study medicine, I was assisted along that path by a wonderful biology teacher. I won't embarrass him by naming him as he is still alive and I remain in touch. He was younger than most of the other teaching staff, but as an 18-year-old Second Lieutenant in the Gloucestershire Regiment on National Service, he had fought in Korea and had witnessed much of his platoon wiped out in an attack by the Chinese Army at the Battle of the Imjin River. No doubt, nowadays he would have been labelled as having had Post-traumatic Stress Disorder (PTSD), and he occasionally had sudden fits of rage, which I am sure we deserved. But he persevered with us, and I was one of three in my year who were lucky enough to gain a place to study medicine at Cambridge.

Nowadays, prospective medical students have to go

through an intimidating set of aptitude tests, which I am quite certain I would never pass. For Cambridge, apart from the A levels, all we needed to do was attend for an interview. I recall being called into a room to face four elderly men (as they seemed to me then) sitting the other side of a large desk. I was offered a glass of sherry, which, as I was only 17 and it was the middle of the afternoon, seemed rather strange. No doubt the fact that I managed not to spill it meant that I had demonstrated an adequate degree of manual dexterity and calmness under pressure. I honestly can't remember any of the questions that I was asked, but several years later I met one of my interviewers and asked him how they chose. 'It's easy,' he explained, 'there's only one question that we pay any attention to and that is, 'Why do you want to study medicine?' If you say that you want to help mankind, or change the world, or cure cancer or anything like that, you are rejected. If you just say that you want to be a doctor, you're in.' It was as simple as that.

The interview process may have been unusual by today's standards but wasn't quite as peculiar as the experience of one of my friends who had applied to read classics. He was called into the tutor's study to find that his interviewer was entirely hidden from view by the pages of *The Times* newspaper. After a prolonged silence, a voice said, 'Impress me.' My quick-witted friend set light to the bottom of the newspaper. It was obviously the correct response as he was admitted with a scholarship, and eventually became a distinguished academic.

In the first three years of our medical studies at Cambridge we did not see a single patient other than the bodies lined up for dissection in the anatomy department, a chilling sight for a naïve teenager. Contact with real people began with my clinical years at Westminster Medical School in London, now sadly closed. In the operating theatres we saw the actual operating table which had been used in 1951 for the removal of a malignant tumour from the lung of King George VI. In fact, the operation had been performed at Buckingham Palace, as, in those days, hospitals came to kings, rather than kings coming to hospitals, but it emphasised to us the principle that everyone should be treated alike. A cleaning lady from Pimlico or a plumber from Vauxhall would be treated with exactly the same care as the monarch.

We were all told the story of the King's operation and how, when the surgeon, Sir Clement Price Thomas,[2] had completed the resection of the tumour, he turned to his registrar, Charles Drew,[3] and instructed him to close the wound. Drew famously protested, 'but it's the King, sir' to which Price Thomas had memorably replied, 'I haven't closed a chest for twenty years and I am not going to practice on the Monarch'. It was an important lesson in the equality of care for which the NHS stood. The hospital was located just down the road from the Houses of Parliament and round the corner from a Salvation Army hostel in Great Peter Street. Finding distinguished MPs and somewhat dishevelled residents of Great Peter Street in neighbouring beds on wards was a regular occurrence. Neither seemed to object, knowing that everyone was given the best care that we could provide.

It is hard nowadays to appreciate the impact of the creation

---

2   Sir Clement Price Thomas KCVO, Consultant Surgeon at Westminster
    Hospital. Like the King he was a heavy smoker and they both died of smoking-
    related diseases.

3   Later a consultant at Westminster Hospital.

of the NHS. For the first time people no longer had to live in fear of illness and wonder whether they could afford care. It is also easy to forget the remarkable changes which have become routine. I remember an elderly relative of my father having an operation for a cataract. Afterwards she had to be nursed on her back in a darkened room for ten days, and could only then see through thick lenses, which allowed quite limited vision. Nowadays, cataracts can be treated with a simple procedure on the same day and perfect visual acuity restored.

When I was newly qualified, patients with heart attacks were treated with several weeks of strict bed rest, while we just waited and hoped for the best. It is now standard practice for patients to be immediately transferred to a specialist cardiology centre for the obstructed blood vessels to be unblocked, with almost miraculous results.

Transplantation, a procedure in which much of the pioneering work had been undertaken at Westminster Hospital, is now almost a matter of routine. A few years ago, I saw a patient in my outpatient clinic who had been referred with a suspected skin cancer. He told me that he had had a heart transplant six years previously. His face looked familiar, and I suddenly realised that just a few months before his visit to my clinic he had been installing a new TV aerial on the roof of my house, climbing up and down a ladder with all his equipment. It seemed little short of a miracle that a man who had been at death's door had been restored to such perfect health, but perhaps the most remarkable thing is the way in which the NHS can treat patients on the basis of their medical needs rather than on their status or wealth.

We have almost come to take for granted safe childbirth and the survival of tiny, premature infants, safe anaesthesia for even for the most complex operations, the virtual elimination of tuberculosis (TB) and the complete eradication of poliomyelitis and diphtheria. I vividly remember a patient telling me how, as a 19-year-old in 1949, he had been diagnosed as having TB. It was a common condition at that time, and frequently fatal. He was sent to a TB sanatorium awaiting an apparently inevitable death, where he stayed for two years, allowed one visitor every six weeks, when suddenly, streptomycin appeared and his life was saved. The list of achievements of the NHS goes on and on, though the human race seems to have a remarkable capacity for generating new problems, such as the epidemic of obesity which ruins so many lives.

I am constantly amazed at some of the changes that I have seen in my own professional lifetime. As a junior doctor, I spent a year working in the cardiology department at Papworth Hospital.[4] It was a rather dilapidated former TB sanatorium, and had not yet achieved the worldwide renown that it has now. Heart pacemakers were, in those days, rather primitive by today's standards, and we still had a small number of patients who had the very first type, called a Lucas induction coil.[5] These patients had had a wire inserted into their hearts, attached to a metal coil placed under their skin. A second coil was taped over the skin attached to a lead, which led to a small box that they

---

4   Now Royal Papworth Hospital in Cambridge.

5   So named because it was designed and built by Joseph Lucas of Birmingham, a long-established firm making electrical parts for cars, in collaboration with a local cardiac surgeon, Leon Abrahams FRCS. The system is described in the paper Treatment of complete heart block with the Lucas induction coil pacemaker, *British Heart Journal* 1971, vol 33:938.

had to carry round with them. The box contained a battery and also a knob that controlled the heart rate. The heart rate was set at 70 beats per minute, but if the patient wanted, for example, to run for a bus, he could turn the rate up to a hundred and then turn it back again once he was safely on board. There was only one serious limiting factor, which was that the batteries only lasted about three weeks and the patient had to come back for a battery change. This was always delegated to the most junior doctor, me, and it certainly caused my own heart to race as I opened the box with a screwdriver and removed the old battery, which caused the patient's heart to stop until I had put the new battery in its place. I lived in fear of having a 'dud' battery but, thankfully, it never happened.[6]

---

6   The implanted batteries, which can last for several years in modern
    pacemakers, were originally designed by the CIA for use in bugging devices
    placed in foreign embassies and the like where, for obvious reasons, replacing
    batteries might not be easy.

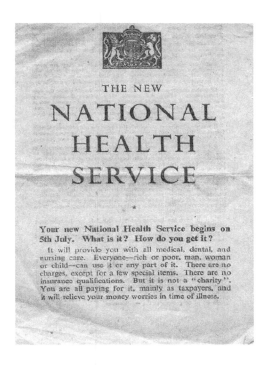

Figure 1. Leaflet explaining the new NHS from 1948.

To some extent the NHS has been a victim of its own success. Patients and their families have come to expect us to perform miracles as a matter of routine, and anyone's death, however inevitable, is regarded as some sort of failure on the part of the medical profession. Sadly, the NHS has, over the years, seen some appalling disasters, sometimes individual ones (as in the Harold Shipman case), and others, corporate failings, as at Stafford Hospital or at Furness General Hospital. Inevitably, human nature being what it is, these cases have cast a cloud of suspicion, which sometimes overshadows the hard work that is done by doctors and nurses every day. But there is a growing feeling in the medical profession that NHS managers, under relentless pressure from their political masters, have all too often been willing to sacrifice quality of care and patient safety in order to meet arbitrary targets. When things go wrong, we all hear a minister or a hospital chief executive saying that 'lessons must be learned', but somehow, they are not. Ministers call for public inquiries and then their reports, diligently compiled, are quietly ignored until the same problems repeat themselves.

From the 1920s onwards, the motor car achieved an iconic status in American culture, a symbol of the independent self-made man with the freedom of the road. But this was accompanied by a catastrophic death toll in road traffic accidents. By the 1960s, some 50,000 people were dying on the roads in the United States each year. In 1965, a young lawyer, Ralph Nader, wrote a book, *Unsafe at Any Speed,* about the American automobile industry and how it was producing cars which, to entice buyers, were visually appealing but inherently dangerous. The industry, incredibly powerful at the time, used all its powers to try to silence him, but the book became a bestseller and deaths on American roads at last began to decline.

In Britain, the NHS has acquired a similar iconic status, a symbol of all that is best in our country, of altruism and of a desire to help those in need. It is almost regarded as bad manners to say anything critical about any part of it. However, I have become increasingly concerned by the way in which I find many doctors are feeling overwhelmed that, in order to practice medicine, they have to fight their way through a bewildering jungle of bureaucracy. At the same time, it appears that there has been a failure to give patient safety the prominence it deserves, and which patients deserve, and that is why I have written this book. I have tried to highlight some of the areas where things have gone wrong. That is not intended as a criticism of the doctors, nurses and others who devote their lives to the NHS, but a reminder that we must not take future success for granted.

Other large organisations, which, for many years, had appalling safety records such as the railways, airlines and the nuclear industry, have transformed themselves. How they did so is nothing short of remarkable, and how it happened has lessons that could be applied to healthcare. Things can change, but there has to be a collective desire to *make* them change. Sadly, the NHS still appears, despite many fine words, not to have prioritised safety. In Chapter 2, I explain how a transformation occurred in the nuclear industry, and the striking contrast in cultures when disaster struck the child of a nuclear worker whilst under the care of the NHS.

CHAPTER 2

Going With a Bang

On 17th October 1956, a young Queen Elizabeth II travelled to a former Second World War ordnance factory in a remote part of Cumbria, near the small village of Seascale. At 12.16 pm precisely, in front of an audience of several thousand people, she pulled the lever which would direct electricity from the world's first nuclear power station, Calder Hall, into the National Grid, where it would supply energy to the town of Workington, some 16 miles down the coast. It was a matter of immense importance to the government, particularly in terms of prestige as Britain slowly emerged from its post-War economic collapse. The ceremony was witnessed by statesmen and scientists from some 40 countries.

In her speech, The Queen said, *'This new power, which has proved itself to be such a terrifying weapon of destruction, is harnessed for the first time for the common good of our community.'* What no one mentioned was that, in fact, the amount of electricity produced by Calder Hall was relatively trivial, and was essentially a by-product of the plutonium production at the adjacent Windscale plant,[7] plutonium being an essential component of a British nuclear deterrent.

---

7   Windscale was subsequently renamed Sellafield.

The British government had initiated a programme of nuclear research in the early part of the Second World War under the code name Tube Alloys, prompted by concerns that Germany was already conducting work aimed at producing an atomic weapon. Two Jewish refugees, Rudolf Peierls and Otto Frisch, who had fled from Germany and Austria respectively, undertook much of the early research at Birmingham University. In 1943, Churchill and Roosevelt signed a secret agreement at a meeting in Quebec, Canada, which allowed sharing of research. Many British scientists who had worked on the Tube Alloys project moved to the United States to work on the *Manhattan Project.* This ultimately led to the dropping of nuclear bombs on the Japanese cities of Hiroshima and Nagasaki in August 1945.

Among the British contingent was a Dane, Niels Bohr, a Nobel prize winner and regarded at the time as the world's foremost expert on nuclear physics, who in 1943, had been smuggled out of Nazi-occupied Denmark by the Danish resistance and brought to Britain. Bohr travelled to the United States under the cover name Nicholas Baker, and made significant contributions, particularly to the design of the detonator mechanism. He did, however, cause some alarm by suggesting that the Allies ought to share their work with the Russians. Roosevelt and Churchill both told him personally that this was not an idea that they wished to pursue.

The two bombs dropped on Japan by the Americans, but with British consent, were named *Little Boy* and *Fat Man* and are estimated to have killed up to a quarter of a million civilians. Thereafter, no one could have been unaware of the horrific destructive potential of nuclear energy.

The British government had assumed that nuclear collaboration would continue after 1945, believing that they had been equal partners in the development of the bomb, but the exposure of two of the British scientific team, Alan May and Klaus Fuchs, as undercover Russian agents, led to the United States banning further co-operation.[8] The detailed information that Fuchs passed to the Russians effectively allowed them to build an atomic weapon without having to spend years on research and development. Faced with the fact that Russia and the USA were now nuclear powers, Clement Attlee, the Labour Prime Minister, decided in 1947 that Britain would have to build its own nuclear weapon if it was not to be marginalised as a world power. To quote Attlee's foreign secretary, Ernest Bevin, 'We've got to have it and it's got to have a bloody Union Jack on it'. It was to this end that the Windscale reactor was built.

It was not long after the discovery of X-rays by the German scientist, William Roentgen, in 1895 that the hazards of radiation began to be recognised. Many of the pioneers in the study of nuclear physics, including Marie Curie and Henri Becquerel, who had jointly been awarded the 1903 Nobel Prize for physics for their discovery of radiation, died themselves

---

8   Klaus Fuchs was another of the German refugee scientists, who had been forced to flee pre-war Germany because of his communist activism, which he kept hidden from the British security services when it came to vetting his suitability for involvement with the project. Unlike most of the German refugees from Nazism he came from a devout Christian family. The defection to Russia of Donald MacLean and Guy Burgess in 1951 created further American suspicions of the British and the security of shared nuclear secrets.

The story of Fuchs' treachery is well described in Professor Frank Close's book *Trinity,* which gives a detailed account of the development of the atomic bomb, but it is not easy reading unless you have at least an A level in physics. Close describes Fuchs as 'The most dangerous spy in history'.

Fuchs' story is also described in Ben MacIntyre's *Agent Sonya.*

from the effects of radiation exposure. One of the few exceptions was Marie Curie's husband, Pierre. He was run over by a bus. Becquerel had earlier made the alarming observation that when he absent-mindedly left a test tube containing radium in his jacket pocket, he developed an ulcer in the underlying area of skin. In Britain, the London Hospital[9] was one of the first to use X-ray to investigate patients. The exposure times in those early days were prolonged; members of the hospital portering team held in place the photographic plates. They all died of the effects of radiation exposure.[10]

Safety issues did not deflect the public enthusiasm for this novel technology. In the 1920s, shoe shops began installing machines in which customers, including children, could observe X-ray images of their feet, in order to check whether their shoes fitted. In the UK they were marketed under the name Pedoscope and in the United States as Foot-o-scope. In Britain it was only after 1958 that it was mandatory for such machines to carry a warning indicating that the radiation was potentially hazardous.

Another popular use of radiation was to paint the dials of watches and clocks with radium in order to make them luminous. The women who did this work[11] were called 'radium girls' and used to lick the tips of their brushes in order to ensure that they had a fine point. Many of them died of radiation-induced mouth cancers or of leukaemia, but the practice

---

9   Now the Royal London.

10   The effect of radiation on the early pioneers is well described in Donald Hunter's 1955 medical textbook 'Diseases of Occupations'.

11   They were all women!

continued until the Second World War when radium was used on the dials fitted in aircraft cockpits. In 1946, when the use of radium paint was finally abandoned, large quantities of radioactive dials from the Timex factory in Dundee were dumped at sea just off the Fife coast, from where they continued to be washed ashore for many years. Until the 1960s, radiation was widely used to treat benign conditions such as acne, warts, hand eczema, ringworm (in young children) and backache. In the early part of my career, I regularly used to see patients who had developed skin cancers as a consequence, even after an interval of 40 or 50 years.

Construction of the nuclear reactors at Windscale began in 1947, and progressed at remarkable speed for an entirely new and potentially hazardous type of technology. No expense was spared, even at a time of post-War austerity, the workers being offered premium wages to work at such a remote and lonely location. The first reactor ('Pile 1') became operational in 1950 and the second ('Pile 2') in 1951. By 1952, enough plutonium had been produced for the first test explosion of a nuclear device *(Operation Hurricane)* in the Monte Bello Islands, located off the northern coast of Western Australia, and thus, on 3rd October 1952, Britain became the world's third nuclear power after the United States and Russia. Whether the bomb, called *Blue Danube,* had Bevin's 'bloody Union Jack' painted on it is not recorded. Over the next six years, 20 further test detonations of a British nuclear weapon were to take place.

From the start, both Windscale Piles were subject to sudden and unexpected temperature rises, which became progressively more alarming and unpredictable as time went on. However, the political imperative was to produce plutonium, and, after

March 1955, when Churchill announced that Britain was to build a hydrogen bomb, tritium[12] and polonium-210,[13] both of which could also be made in the Windscale reactors.

In the summer of 1955, environmental tests had discovered evidence of radioactive uranium oxide near the Windscale site, and further evidence of radioactive leakage was found in January 1957. In July 1957, abnormally high levels of radioactive strontium-90 were found in milk from neighbouring farms, but nothing was to be allowed to impede the progress of the manufacture of vital materials for Britain's nuclear weaponry. This was of particular importance as Britain and the USA were negotiating a renewal of their nuclear co-operation. Any perceived deficiencies in the British nuclear programme would potentially weaken its position.

The scientists had been repeatedly expressing their concerns over the safety situation, but they were ignored by politicians and the military, who were totally focused on the need for materials for atomic weaponry. 'They were running much too close to the precipice', said one scientist from the nuclear research laboratory at Harwell.

Then in the autumn of 1957, just a year after The Queen's triumphant visit, disaster struck. On 7th October 1957, abnormal temperature measurements were noted in Pile 1, and by 9th October it was obvious that something was seriously wrong. Various manoeuvres were undertaken to attempt to cool the

---

12 A radioactive isotope of hydrogen with an atomic weight of three.
13 A highly unstable radioactive element used to trigger the chain reaction in nuclear weapons. Polonium was the element used by the Russians to murder Alexander Litvinenko in London, in 2006.

Pile, but by the 10th October it was clear that there was a fire in the reactor, and that radioactive material was dispersing from the chimney into the atmosphere.

The hero of the hour was the duty manager on the site, Tom Tuohy. He faced a horrific situation, and as he said afterwards, 'Mankind had never faced a situation like this; there's no-one to give you any advice'. He added, 'I never thought about my own safety. I just knew there were things I could do, and I got on and did them'. All the standard methods of cooling the Pile had failed, and if it were allowed to just burn, radiation would spread over a large swathe of North West England, potentially causing the area to become uninhabitable for a century.

Tuohy decided, after several highly perilous inspections of the site, to flood the reactor with water. This was against all conventional advice as, theoretically, it might have triggered an explosion, but allowing the reactor to just burn itself out was simply not an option. His intuition was right, and there was no explosion. His personal bravery was extraordinary. 'I went up to check several times until I was satisfied that the fire was out. I did stand to one side, sort of hopefully, but if you're staring straight at the core of a shutdown reactor, you're going to get quite a bit of radiation'.

Although the release of radiation from Windscale was only about 1% of that which subsequently occurred after Chernobyl,[14] radiation was detected over an extensive area of Northern Europe. There was no immediate loss of life, and a

14   The precise number of deaths resulting from the accident at Chernobyl is still a matter of debate.

retrospective review of Windscale workers many years later showed no excess of deaths from cancer or other radiation-related diseases. An analysis of the recorded radiation levels in the area would indicate that about 200 extra cases of cancer would have arisen over time. As a precaution, the consumption of milk produced in the surrounding 200 square miles was banned, and large quantities were diluted and poured into the Irish Sea (to the considerable annoyance of the Irish government).

Harold Macmillan, the Prime Minister, was anxious to impress on the public that there was no cause for concern, and on the Americans that the problem was caused by mistakes by technicians on site, rather than any intrinsic flaw in British technology. He was desperate that the Americans would not find a pretext to abandon the mutual defence agreement, which was, in fact, signed in early 1958.

A board of inquiry was set up immediately after the fire under Sir William Penney (later Lord Penney). Penney had a deep understanding of nuclear issues, having been the leader of the British group in the Manhattan Project, and having supervised the detonation of the first British atomic bomb in 1952. However, Penney could hardly have been regarded as independent, being the head of the weapons division of the UK Atomic Energy Authority (UKAEA), and later, the organisation's Chairman.

Penney's report, produced in less than three weeks, put the entire blame for the fire on errors by the site technicians, a conclusion which was remarkably convenient from Macmillan's point of view. The fact that a major national catastrophe had only been avoided by a fluke, together with Tom Tuohy's selfless bravery, seems to have been completely overlooked, or at the very least, hidden from the public and the Americans.

Tom Tuohy emerged physically unscathed from what must have been a considerable personal exposure to radiation (he had removed his radiation protection badge before inspecting the Pile), and lived to the age of 90. When later asked what he thought of the British officials who had told their American counterparts that the fire had been caused by the negligence of the Windscale staff, he is reported to have said, 'I thought they were a shower of bastards'. His work colleagues felt that he did not receive the recognition that he deserved.[15]

Whatever the government's public position over the causes and consequences of the Windscale fire, they and the whole nuclear industry were shocked by how close they had come to disaster. Also, the public had suddenly become much more aware of the potential implications of nuclear accidents, and many became, quite understandably, sceptical of government reassurance. The Campaign for Nuclear Disarmament (CND) was founded in November 1957, with the philosopher, Bertrand Russell, as its president, and the author, JB Priestley, as a prominent supporter. It held its first public meeting in February 1958.

A more detailed inquiry into the events at Windscale was established in January 1958 under Sir Alexander Fleck, the chairman of Imperial Chemical Industries (ICI). Fleck had a background in physics and had, in his early career, been involved

---

15   He received a CBE for 'services to the nuclear industry' in 1969.

in radiation research. In his years at ICI, he had developed an excellent grasp of running complex and potentially dangerous manufacturing sites, including the production of explosives. He was also a firm believer in the idea, somewhat unfashionable at the time, of managers listening to their staff, with the result that ICI had always maintained excellent industrial relations, not a common scenario in British industry in the 1950s.

There was a clear need for a radical review of nuclear safety. The system of ignoring warning signs and 'hoping for the best' simply couldn't continue. The situation was made more urgent by the construction having begun in 1957 of four new nuclear power stations at Berkeley in Gloucestershire, Bradwell in Essex, Hunterston in Ayrshire and Hinkley Point in Somerset. Chapelcross, on the Scottish border near Gretna, which was modelled on Calder Hall and which produced electricity as a by-product of atomic weapon production, had begun construction in 1955 and came on stream in 1959.

These projects marked the real beginning of civil nuclear power generation in the United Kingdom (as opposed to electricity production as a by-product of nuclear weapon manufacture), which has been supported, with various levels of enthusiasm, by both the Labour and Conservative parties ever since. Margaret Thatcher's government was particularly enthusiastic, believing that nuclear energy would be an antidote to industrial unrest in the coal industry and to Middle East oil embargoes. At its peak in 1997, nuclear energy provided 27% of Britain's electricity. It still accounts for about 19%, but clearly, and especially after the Windscale fire, safety would have to take precedence if there was to be public acceptance. Further pressure was applied in April 1959 when news began to leak out of Russia of an even larger nuclear incident in Siberia in September 1958.[16]

Fleck's report focused on the organisational changes that would need to be deployed to ensure future nuclear safety. His recommendations were adopted by the government and came into law under the Nuclear Installations Act (1959). One of the key elements of this was the creation of the Nuclear Installations Inspectorate (NII), which was responsible for all matters relating to nuclear safety and that the NII should be totally separate from the UKAEA, which at the time was in charge of the entire nuclear programme in Britain.

This model of making the body responsible for safety, independent of those who run nuclear installations, was essentially the same as was subsequently adopted on the railway network and the oil and gas industry, and ensured that economic pressures or commercial convenience could not be allowed to compromise the overriding need for safety.

The success of the NII can be measured by the fact that in the 60 years since it came into operation, there has not been a single external radiation leak from a UK nuclear power generation site. This represents a complete transformation from the early days of the Windscale operation. The NII is responsible, not just for the safety of the everyday running of nuclear sites, but also for the whole process of design, commissioning and construction, including ensuring that

---

16 The incident occurred at a plutonium production site in the closed city of Ozyorsk, not even marked on maps. The precise details remain obscure, but it is ranked third behind Chernobyl and Fukushima on the International Nuclear and Radiological Event Scale (INES) list of nuclear disasters.

suppliers and subcontractors fully understand and comply with their responsibilities. The fundamental belief is that nuclear facilities must run safely or not at all.

Clearly, the nuclear industry has the potential for disasters on quite a different scale from any other, so the consequences of every hazard, however improbable, are carefully assessed. There has even been evaluation of the risks of earthquakes and tsunamis. The last tsunami to hit Britain was in 1755, after the Lisbon earthquake, and one is thought to have hit the east coast of Scotland around 6500 BC. A meteorite strike is the risk that most concerns the NII, which places in perspective how safe they believe our nuclear power stations are.

Earthquakes, tsunamis and meteorites may seem fairly improbable hazards, but the safety systems in the nuclear industry have been proven effective in some unlikely situations. For instance, in June 2011, the nuclear reactor at Torness on the North Sea coast some 30 miles from Edinburgh, had to be temporarily shut down when the sea water used to cool the system was found to contain huge numbers of jellyfish and there was a risk of the filters becoming blocked. The safety procedure went smoothly and there was no danger of a radiation leak. In the same year, an Atlantic grey seal, chasing fish, became trapped in the water inflow system at Hinkley Point; again, the system coped and the seal was unharmed.

But perhaps the most striking illustration of how the nuclear industry has tackled safety, in a way that the NHS has conspicuously failed to do, is the sad story of Joshua Titcombe.

Joshua was born on 27th October 2008 at the maternity

department of Furness General Hospital in Barrow-in-Furness, a hospital that was part of the Morecambe Bay Hospitals NHS Trust. His father, James Titcombe, was a project manager at the Sellafield nuclear site a little further up the Cumbria coast. Joshua was delivered after an apparently normal pregnancy. His mother's waters had broken a few days beforehand, but she had been advised by the midwives not to come into hospital until labour was established. Everything seemed fine to the delighted parents, but a few hours later Joshua's mother developed a high fever, abdominal pain and collapsed. She required treatment with intravenous fluids and antibiotics, presumably having developed an infection as a result of the prolonged rupture of membranes, subsequently confirmed by microbiological tests. The Titcombes queried whether Joshua himself should be checked for infection, but they were reassured. In fact, his temperature was below normal, which, in a neonate, is a serious warning sign of sepsis, but his parents were again told that nothing was wrong. Something clearly was not right, but it was not until the next day when Joshua was severely unwell that the paediatricians were called.

Joshua was transferred as an emergency to Manchester for more specialist care and then to Newcastle in a last-ditch effort to save his life, where a new form of treatment called ECMO (extracorporeal membrane oxygenation) was available. Sadly, Joshua died on 5th November 2008, aged nine days, of overwhelming sepsis and a lung haemorrhage. His parents were heartbroken.

After Joshua's death, the distraught Titcombes sought some explanation, but were initially told that it was just an unfortunate occurrence and a 'one-off'. James Titcombe, who in his working life in the nuclear industry had been steeped in the culture of openness and blame-free enquiry into safety incidents, was left feeling utterly bemused. Mysteriously, within a month of his death, the care records for Joshua's admission had disappeared, never to be found,[17] but it was clear that what had happened to Joshua was not a unique case. There had been a string of catastrophes and near misses on the maternity unit dating back to at least 2004. Earlier, in 2008, one of the consultant obstetricians had written to the medical director of the hospital trust expressing his concerns about the care given to a baby who had died during labour and drawing comparisons with a similar incident in 2004. He warned that further tragedies would occur unless remedial action was taken. There was no response to the letter and no action appeared to follow.

In early 2010, the hospital commissioned an external report under Professor Dame Pauline Fielding into the maternity services. The report suggested that the five serious incidents in 2008 were unconnected, but had lowered staff morale. There was no real suggestion that there was anything more amiss. At this time, the Morecambe Bay Hospitals Trust was applying for 'Foundation Trust status,'[18] and Furness Hospital was subject to an unannounced inspection by the Care Quality Commission (CQC). It was duly given a clean bill of health, and the regulatory body, Monitor, awarded the hospital group Foundation Trust

---

17   Missing records do not seem unique to the NHS. In September 2020, the Grenfell Tower Inquiry heard that e-mails, documents and design drawings relating to the Grenfell Tower refurbishment had been lost (https://www.itv.com/news/london/2020-09-14/grenfell-files-lost-forever-after-laptop-wiped-inquiry-hears). Vital prosecution documents also went missing in the murder trial of Dr John Bodkin Adams (see Chapter 5, *The Trial of the Century*).

18   See Chapter 9, 'Stafford' for an explanation of Foundation Trusts.

status in October 2010.

Immediately after the CQC visit, James Titcombe wrote to Andrew Lansley, the Secretary of State for Health, urging him to look at Furness General Hospital and warning him that other lives were at risk. He received no reply from the minister, who instead instructed an official at the Department of Health's 'customer service centre' to inform Mr Titcombe that he was 'unable to comment.'

Initially, the Newcastle coroner (Joshua had died in Newcastle, so the case had fallen under that jurisdiction), rejected the Titcombe family's request for an inquest, but in 2011 an inquest was finally held in Cumbria into Joshua's death. The coroner determined that Joshua had died of a pneumococcal infection, the same organism that had affected his mother, and that there was an 80% chance that the timely administration of antibiotics would have saved him. The coroner was critical of failures by the hospital to recognise or act on the symptoms of infection, to listen to the concerns of the parents, and to maintain adequate records. He also found a 'strained and dysfunctional relationship between the midwives and the paediatricians' and was concerned at the apparent collusion of the eleven midwives who gave evidence. He further noted that 'incriminating' notes containing observations about Joshua's condition might well have been deliberately destroyed.

At the same time, the Cumbria police announced that they were starting an investigation into several deaths on the maternity unit at Furness General Hospital. Fifteen officers were allocated to the case. In the end, no arrests were made or prosecutions brought, but in 2012 the police announced that they were passing their concerns to the Nursing and Midwifery Council (NMC), the regulatory body responsible for disciplinary matters in the midwifery and nursing professions. In the event, the NMC did not take any action until 2014 and the last hearings into those involved in Joshua Titcombe's care only took place in 2017, eight years after his death. Midwives under investigation continued to practice and, in some cases, were involved in subsequent serious incidents involving avoidable harm and death. At the same time, the NMC spent some £240,000 on legal fees trying to withhold information from Joshua's father. It was only in 2019 that the NMC finally apologised to him.

In May 2011, the BBC broadcast a *Panorama* documentary about the systematic abuse of patients in Winterbourne View, Gloucestershire, a private facility for young adults with severe learning disabilities and autism. Both Castlebeck, the company that owned the care home and the CQC, the body mentioned earlier which has the statutory duty to regulate and inspect healthcare facilities, had ignored pleas from a senior nurse at Winterbourne View to take action.[19]

The Chief Executive of the CQC, Cynthia Bower, resigned, and her successor ordered an independent inquiry into the organisation by the management consultants, Grant Thornton. As part of their inquiry, they received evidence from a whistle-blower within the CQC that the 2010 report into the maternity service at Furness General Hospital had apparently been

---

19   In 2012, six members of staff at Winterbourne View were sent to prison and five others were given suspended prison sentences. The average weekly fee for a patient was £3500. Castlebeck Care (Teesdale) Ltd went into administration but no action was taken against any of its senior executives.

'doctored' so as not to show the hospital in a bad light, which would have impeded the Trust's application for Foundation status. The new Chairman of the CQC admitted that the organisation was 'not fit for purpose', and in 2013, the Health Secretary, Jeremy Hunt (who had replaced Andrew Lansley, the minister who had ignored James Titcombe's earlier warnings) ordered a full, independent inquiry into the deaths on the maternity unit at Furness General Hospital. In September 2013, the CQC, in a remarkable turnaround, appointed James Titcombe to a position as national adviser on quality and safety; 'I want to help ensure we get patient safety and culture right', he said.

In the same year, the Health Service Ombudsman, Dame Julie Mellor, upheld three complaints that the Titcombes had made against what was now called the University Hospitals of Morecambe Bay NHS Foundation Trust, and said that change was needed 'from the ward to the board' and the Trust's lack of honesty in handling complaints had caused the family 'unnecessary pain and further distress'. She apologised for her predecessor having refused to investigate the Titcombes' original complaint made in 2010.

At last, James Titcombe's dogged determination to seek the truth was beginning to bear fruit. The meticulous application of the safety principles he had learned in the nuclear industry had triumphed over initial rejections from the Trust, the Newcastle coroner, the Health Service Ombudsman, the CQC and the Health Secretary.

Hunt's inquiry was led by Dr Bill Kirkup, who had previously been a member of the Hillsborough Independent Panel, which had investigated the disaster at Hillsborough Stadium in Sheffield on 15th April 1989 in which 96 football fans had been crushed to death. He had also conducted an inquiry into the activities of Jimmy Savile at Broadmoor Hospital. His report into the events at Furness General Hospital, published in 2015, described a 'lethal mix' of failures that had led to the unnecessary deaths of 11 babies and one mother, and called the avoidable incidents 'serious and shocking'.

It also criticised the wider NHS for the way it had monitored and regulated the hospital, or rather, had failed to regulate and monitor it. There had been 'simultaneous failures of a great many systems at almost every level, from labour ward to headquarters of national bodies'. Jeremy Hunt, speaking in the House of Commons, described the situation as 'a second Mid Staffs'. He was referring to the catastrophic situation at Stafford Hospital, run by the Mid Staffordshire NHS Foundation Trust, where it is estimated that several hundred people may have died through inadequate and negligent care, as had been revealed by the report of Robert Francis QC in 2013.[20]

In the conclusion to Dr Kirkup's maternity services report, he raised the question as to whether the same situation might arise at other hospitals in the NHS. He adds, 'It is vital to learn all of the lessons so as to improve every layer of the system and eliminate the defects. If we were foolish enough to rely on the unlikelihood of the defects becoming aligned again in this way, sooner or later they would, with tragic and unnecessary repetition'.

---

20   See Chapter 9 'Stafford'.

In the same year as the Kirkup report was published, James Titcombe was awarded an OBE for services to patient safety, but sadly, it wasn't long before evidence began to emerge that Furness General Hospital was not a 'one-off'.

By 2017, stories began to appear of an even larger maternity scandal, this time at the Shrewsbury and Telford Hospital NHS Trust. Dozens of babies had died over the years, and many more had suffered catastrophic injuries. The Healthcare Commission (the forerunner of the CQC) had been aware of the problems since 2007. By 2020, evidence of the scale of the problem was still emerging, and a police inquiry was in progress. The numbers of those potentially involved continue to expand.

James Titcombe, who had devoted years of his life trying to bring about change, noted, 'This is more evidence that the NHS needs to face up to the fact that there has been a systemic problem in maternity services. Yet again it has taken families to be the catalyst to get this exposed.'[21]

Nor, distressingly, is the situation at Shrewsbury and Telford unique. Whilst the coronavirus epidemic has been the main focus of the NHS and the press in 2020, further catastrophic maternity care failings have been emerging in Kent, at the Queen Elizabeth the Queen Mother Hospital, Margate, run by the East Kent Hospitals University NHS Foundation Trust; in Essex, at Basildon University Hospital, run by Basildon and Thurrock University NHS Foundation Trust; at Barnstable in

---

21   James Titcombe's account of events is recorded in his 2015 book 'Joshua's Story: Uncovering the Morecambe Bay NHS Scandal'.

North Devon and at two hospitals in South Wales. In all these cases, although the full facts have yet to emerge, the stories bear a striking similarity to the tragedies that befell babies and their parents at Furness General Hospital.

In February 2020, Jeremy Hunt, who in his role as Health Secretary, had in 2013, established the independent inquiry into maternity services at Furness General Hospital and was appointed Chairman of the House of Commons Select Committee on Health and Social Care (HSCC). One of his first actions was to call for a public inquiry into maternity care, in the light of these continuing scandals. In September 2020, he revealed that in the financial year 2018-2019, the cost to the NHS of compensation and litigation relating to NHS maternity units, was £954 million.[22] As Mr Hunt wrote in the *Daily Mail*, 'Something has gone seriously wrong', adding, 'We have appallingly high levels of avoidable harm and death in our healthcare system. In healthcare we seem to just accept it as inevitable'. Meanwhile, Bill Kirkup, who undertook the inquiry at Furness General Hospital, is now undertaking a similar inquiry into the maternity services in East Kent, and will no doubt discover repeated failings that he previously identified.

At Furness General Hospital alone, compensation in 37 cases came to £45 million. But quite apart from the financial costs, each case of unnecessary and avoidable harm is a tragedy for the whole family, with the death of a mother or of a new-born baby or a child with lifelong handicap through brain injury. And the suffering of the families is further aggravated by the time it takes for compensation claims to be settled. The largest

---

22 £954 million equates to almost £2000 for every child born in the UK.

claim at Furness, relating to a child born with catastrophic brain damage and requiring constant lifelong care, took 12 years of litigation. The effect on the family in having to care for a child and battle through the courts must have been unimaginable.

Joshua Titcombe's story shows the vivid contrast between the nuclear industry, where a single 'near miss' in 1957 was enough to produce a lasting cultural change, and the NHS, which seems to lurch relentlessly from one catastrophe to the next. Clearly, Mr Hunt has got the message,[23] but sadly, too many others have not.

---

23 Jeremy Hunt served as Secretary of State for Health for seven years, the longest holder of the office, and is now Chairman of the Parliamentary Committee on Health. He is therefore one of the very few politicians who has shown a long-term interest in health matters.

CHAPTER 3

Crash Landing

On 17th December 1903, two bicycle mechanics from Dayton, Ohio, Wilbur and Orville Wright, stood on a remote beach near the small town of Kitty Hawk, North Carolina, and took turns in propelling a rather curious kite-like structure that they called the *Wright Flyer,* into the air. It was powered by a twelve-horsepower engine, which, by means of a bicycle chain, turned the propeller. At the fourth attempt the contraption flew nearly 300 yards in just under a minute. A lone photographer was present to record for posterity the moment that powered human flight became a reality.

Interest in this new technology was immediate. In 1908, Wilbur Wright came to Europe and his flying demonstrations attracted enormous crowds. In 1909, the proprietor of the *Daily Mail*, Lord Northcliffe, offered a prize of £1000 for the first person to fly across the English Channel. He had hoped that the Wright brothers would accept the challenge, but Orville was recovering from serious injuries sustained in a crash and Wilbur was unwilling to do it on his own. Also, he did not need the money as he had amassed a fortune giving flying displays. On 25th July 1909, the Frenchman, Louis Blériot, achieved that very feat, arriving from France in just over 30 minutes. Remarkably, his plane was not even equipped with a compass and at one point he got lost in a cloud![24]

The early days of flying were highly dangerous. Charles Rolls, the co-founder with Henry Royce of the Rolls-Royce company, was the first person to die in an aeroplane accident in Britain (and the tenth in the world), crashing a *Wright Flyer* at a flying display in Bournemouth in 1910. Ironically, he had also been the first person to be issued with an 'Aviator Certificate' by the Royal Aero Club (RAeC) earlier the same year.

The military potential of flying soon became obvious, and the Royal Flying Corps (RFC) was established in May 1912 (its counterpart the Royal Naval Air Corps was created in 1914, and the two units amalgamated to form the Royal Air Force in 1918). The RFC's first fatal crash occurred just a few weeks after its creation. An order was issued after the crash stating 'Flying will continue this evening as usual', thus beginning a tradition.

In May 1913, a popular and experienced RFC pilot, Desmond Arthur, was killed in an aeroplane accident near the RFC flying school near Montrose, Scotland.[25] A wing of his plane had snapped off in mid-air. A report by the Accidents and Investigation Committee of the RAeC attributed the crash to a previous faulty repair, but a government inquiry blamed pilot error. Quite what sort of error would make a wing fall off was not explained. Controversy and the case rumbled on, and the general technical deficiencies of aircraft maintenance were repeatedly raised in parliament, but, as with the NHS in more

---

24 The 1965 film *Those Magnificent Men in their Flying Machines* was largely based on the story of Lord Northcliffe's challenge.

25 Scotland's first flying fatality.

recent years, it was easier and more convenient to blame the individual than the system. Arthur seems to have had a curious posthumous revenge, because sightings of his ghost flying over Scotland were seen for many years and on one occasion this resulted in an RAF plane making an emergency landing.

This tendency to blame the pilot was not just a British habit. The US Army bought a number of aircraft from the Wright brothers in 1912 and 1913. All of them crashed with fatal outcomes and, although there had been six consecutive instances of the planes suddenly and inexplicably nosediving, the Wrights insisted that it all must have been down to pilot error. Blériot and the Wright brothers were very rare examples of early aviation pioneers who were not themselves killed in accidents. It was analogous to the pioneers of X-ray, most of whom had died from excessive radiation exposure.

The First World War saw a great expansion in aviation activity and considerable technical improvement. Nearly 10,000 RFC airmen died in the War, some being killed in combat, but many others in flying mishaps, however, these numbers were dwarfed by the enormous military losses on the ground. 'Flying aces', a term officially applied to those known to have made five or more kills, became household names, and some, such as Albert Ball, Billy Bishop and 'Mick' Mannock, were national heroes. There was a rather curious chivalry in air combat, and even enemy pilots such as Manfred von Richthofen ('The Red Baron') were held in awe. It was very different from the anonymity of the carnage of the ground war, although inevitably, most of the aces died in combat.

In fact, the RFC had established an Accidents Investigation

Branch of its own in 1915 under an 'Inspector of Accidents' Captain George Cockburn. Cockburn was awarded an OBE at the end of the war, but with the frequency of incidents it is doubtful it would have been possible for the majority of crashes to be subject to any sort of detailed scrutiny.

The inherent danger of aviation did not discourage public interest in flying or provoke much interest in safety, and no doubt, young pilots who had survived the War must have felt almost invincible. But aeroplanes remained dangerous. The first airline company in Britain, Air Transport and Travel Ltd,[26] suffered four crashes in its first year of operation, this included their first commercial flight from Hendon in North West London to Bournemouth in May 1919. This was just a month before Alcock and Brown made their first non-stop transatlantic flight which finished with a crash-landing in a boggy field in the West of Ireland. They were acclaimed as national heroes and knighted by King George V a few days later, but within a few months Alcock had died in a crash *en route* to an air show in France.

Airmail was also developing in a rudimentary fashion. The French company *L'Aéropostale*, which eventually turned into *Air France,* was a pioneer in this field. It had so many crashes in the 1920s and 30s that the postal authorities in France produced a special hand-stamp to frank letters damaged in air accidents. Examples of these postmarks still turn up from time to time in stamp auctions and are highly prized by philatelists. By 1939, commercial flying, whether of passengers or freight,

---

26 The company was a subsidiary of Airco, an aeroplane manufacturing company, whose chief designer was Geoffrey de Havilland.

was still happening on a fairly modest scale, and while most people would have *seen* an aeroplane, few would have actually *flown* in one.

Aeroplanes had been rather a sideshow in the First World War, but in the Second they were very much centre stage, their role enhanced by major technical developments including RADAR[27] and the jet engine. Aeroplanes became larger, faster, more robust and capable of carrying much heavier loads. Sadly, there were many more crashes and deaths of crews. In the Second World War, RAF Bomber Command alone lost over 8,000 planes and over 55,000 men. Again, it was rarely possible to determine how many crashes were caused by defects in the aircraft or avoidable human factors rather than by enemy action, and it is doubtful whether much systematic effort was made to investigate.

By the end of the war, flying, although still inherently dangerous, had become considerably safer. Planes were of more robust construction, and had more powerful engines, the greater speed adding to their stability. Radio allowed improved communication of weather conditions, and planes were equipped with better instrumentation. But in civilian flight, larger planes meant greater potential loss of life.

The greatest of all of the technical developments, and the one that paved the way for mass civil air transport, was the jet engine. In parallel, both the British, using the designs of Sir Frank Whittle, and the Germans, had been working on

---

27   RADAR is an acronym of RAdio Detection And Ranging.

jet propulsion of aircraft, with the Gloster Meteor[28] and the Messerschmitt Me 262 entering service almost simultaneously in early 1944. At the end of the war, the possibility of applying these new, more efficient and powerful engines to civilian planes was obvious and the de Havilland company at Hatfield was the first to seize the opportunity.

On 2nd May 1952, a de Havilland Comet operated by British Overseas Airways Corporation (BOAC) undertook the world's first commercial jet flight from London to Johannesburg, and in August of the same year, Prince Philip, always an enthusiast for new technology, flew by Comet from Helsinki, where he had been watching the Olympic Games. Jet engines resulted in a dramatic reduction in flight time[29] and improved comfort, and were an immediate commercial success. In June 1953, Queen Elizabeth the Queen Mother and Princess Margaret travelled on a special Comet flight as guests of the company. As with the Queen's visit to the Calder Hall nuclear power station, the royal family never allowed their personal safety to get in the way of promoting British technology, for by this time, Comets had already started to demonstrate an alarming tendency to crash.

In October 1952, a BOAC Comet had failed to take off from the runway in Rome. There were only two injuries, but the plane was a write-off. In March 1953, there was an almost identical incident at Karachi, with 11 fatalities, this time the aircraft

---

28   Gloster aeroplanes were so called because they were originally built in Gloucestershire, but the origins of the spelling are unclear. Gloster Aircraft Limited was taken over by Hawker in the 1930s, and subsequently became Hawker Siddeley.

29   The Comet flight from London to Tokyo took 36 hours compared to 86 hours for its conventionally powered rivals.

belonging to a Canadian airline. In both cases, pilot error was blamed but there were strong suspicions amongst senior BOAC pilots, ultimately vindicated, that there was something wrong with the design. De Havilland subsequently reconfigured the profile of the leading edge of the wings, which improved the lift on take-off.

In May 1953, another BOAC Comet crashed shortly after take-off from Calcutta in a thunder squall, with the loss of all 43 people on board. Eye witnesses spoke of the plane coming down without its wings. Investigations concluded that the crash had been the result of a combination of the weather and pilot error. Again, quite what sort of pilot error and weather conditions make an aeroplane's wings fall off was not explained.

The chief Comet test pilot, Group Captain Johnny 'Cat's Eyes' Cunningham, pronounced that there was nothing wrong with the planes. Cunningham had earned a considerable reputation during the Battle of Britain, and had become something of a celebrity akin to the World War One flying aces. He had been given the nickname 'Cat's Eyes' by the press to explain his remarkable record of kills at night, attributing these to his visual acuity rather than to RADAR, which was still a secret at the time. His comments about the Comet probably carried an element of bravado. There was clearly something fundamentally wrong but it was easier to blame the pilots and hope for the best than to address the underlying issues. It almost seemed that the aviation industry was still in denial, with the mindset of the pioneering days of the RFC, and its order 'Flying will continue this evening as usual'.

Things went from bad to worse in 1954. In January of that

year, a BOAC Comet, taking off from Rome (the site of an earlier Comet crash), *en route* to London on the final leg of a flight from Singapore, crashed into the sea near the island of Elba. There were no witnesses and radio communication had been abruptly lost. All 35 people on board died. BOAC grounded their fleet of Comets immediately and an inquiry began. The local pathologist examined bodies that had been retrieved and said that they all showed identical injuries suggestive of acute decompression, and that they had all died before the plane hit the water; in other words, there had been sudden loss of cabin pressure in mid-air. The official inquiry, which gave its conclusions before efforts had been completed to reconstruct and test the wreckage, came to no clear conclusion. With the government aware of the importance of the Comet project to the aerospace industry, it pressed BOAC to resume flying, which they did within two months of the crash, and with many questions unanswered.

Less than three weeks after the Comet returned to service, in April 1954, a Comet, chartered to South African Airways took off from Rome (again) bound for Cairo, as a leg on a journey from London to Johannesburg. The plane crashed into the Mediterranean near Naples with the loss of all 21 crew and passengers. The Comet's certificate of airworthiness (CoA) was revoked and the whole Comet fleet grounded. De Havilland and the Royal Aircraft Establishment (RAE) conducted a detailed investigation and their conclusion was that the Comet had an inherent weakness of the cabin structure. In part, this related to the square portholes, the corners of which were particular points of weakness. De Havilland undertook a complete re-design of the fuselage, including replacing the square portholes,[30] but although the Comet returned to service in October 1958, this last crash was the end of the plane as a serious economic proposition. The Boeing 707 and the Douglas DC-9 were already at an advanced stage for their launch and thus became the market leaders. One can only speculate how different it would have been if only the first incidents had been inspected with the rigour that is now expected and applied to aircraft safety, rather than reverting to the traditional tendency to blame the pilots, who all too often were not in a position to defend themselves, not to mention the extraordinary loss of life.

BOAC was still not out of the woods. With the Comet out of action, the aeroplane of choice for long-distance civilian flying was the Boeing 377 Stratocruiser. Unfortunately, it was yet another plane with a dreadful safety record that was involved in numerous incidents, but this deterred neither the airline nor the regulatory authorities on either side of the Atlantic. With so many senior officials in aviation both in Britain and the USA having air force backgrounds, the attitude of 'the show must go on' still held sway. On Christmas Day 1954, a BOAC Stratocruiser crashed at Prestwick Airport in Scotland with the loss of 28 lives. It was only when the Stratocruiser was superseded by the Boeing 707 and the DC-9 that its era of mayhem ended, as a result of its lack of utility rather than its alarming tendency to crash.

In February 1958, members of the Manchester United football team, including a young Bobby Charlton,[31] were

---

30   I had always wondered why aeroplane windows are round.

31   Later Sir Bobby Charlton.

returning from a European Cup match in Belgrade. Their plane had stopped in Munich to refuel and crashed on take-off in icy conditions. Eight of the team, including 21-year-old Duncan Edwards, the rising star of English football, were killed, along with others on the flight including the pilot. The Germans demonstrated that it was not just the British aviation authorities who had a tendency to blame the pilot, claiming that he had failed to de-ice the wings of the plane. In fact, he had, but the airport had failed to adequately de-ice the runway, with fatal results. The pilot was posthumously cleared of blame in 1968, no doubt to the relief of his family and colleagues.

Larger aeroplanes meant more fatalities. In June 1972, a British European Airways Trident crashed near Staines shortly after take-off, killing all 118 people on board. It was, at the time, the deadliest air accident in United Kingdom history.[32]

Since 1987, the investigation team have been called the Air Accidents Investigation Branch (AAIB), previously Accidents Investigation Branch (AIB) and they investigated the crash, as was normal procedure at the time. However, Michael Heseltine, who had just been appointed 'Minister for Aerospace', a new role within the Department of Trade and Industry (DTI), ordered a Board of Inquiry be set up. He was entitled to do this if he considered there was a serious matter of public interest, which this clearly was as such a large loss of life cast a pall over the whole aviation industry. No-one wanted a repeat of the Comet fiasco, which had not only cost lives but had caused

---

32 The Lockerbie bombing of Pan Am Flight 103 on December 1988 is generally not recorded as an accident as it was a criminal act of terrorism; 270 people died, including 11 on the ground.

severe economic damage to the aerospace industry and to British technological prestige.

Having two separate inquiries was, in retrospect, not a success. The professional crash investigators of the AAIB took, as their remit, establishing the facts. The inquiry took a more legalistic approach, and some of the American lawyers, representing families of the deceased, took a very aggressive approach in their cross-examination of expert witnesses of a type which may have been familiar on American courtroom TV dramas but which had not been seen in a British court. One of the AAIB expert investigators found the stress so overwhelming that he committed suicide. The approach did not prove to be a satisfactory way of working out what had really happened and which of the various issues identified was crucial in causing the disaster.

What *was* established was that the Trident had a tendency to stall on take-off, that the plane was right on the upper limit of its permitted payload, and that the Captain had had a furious argument in the crew room before take-off and was seen to go white with rage.[33] It was found at postmortem that the Captain was found to have had a heart attack shortly before the crash. The Second Officer (the co-pilot, who would have been expected to take control if the Captain was incapacitated) had been relatively inexperienced.

Perhaps what was most helpfully established was that

---

33 I have always told my children that they must never drive if they had just had an argument; researching the story of the Staines air disaster has reinforced my view on this.

muddled and competing inquiries do not reach the truth and, fortunately, this set in motion a re-organisation of how air crashes are investigated in the UK, which in turn has transformed air safety. Accidents and serious incidents[34] are investigated independently to establish the facts, and not to apportion blame, with review of previous similar incidents and with recommendations as to what lessons can be learned. The object is for safety improvement, and their independence ensures that conclusions are not influenced by commercial or political factors, as had clearly happened in the past. As mentioned, the AAIB came about and as such, other analogous bodies were set up for the railways and the shipping industry.

The effectiveness of this approach was demonstrated by the Manchester air disaster of 1985, after which the recommendations of the investigation transformed the internal design of civilian aeroplanes worldwide. It is probably not a coincidence that British Airways (BA) has not been involved in a single accident fatality in the subsequent 35 years, and that neither Ryanair (established 1985), nor EasyJet plc (established 1995), have ever had an accident fatality. There has been no fatal commercial passenger air crash in the United Kingdom since the Kegworth air disaster of 1989. It was simply an extraordinary transformation.

The Manchester air disaster involved a Boeing 737 operated by British Airtours, a subsidiary of BA, full of holidaymakers *en route* to Corfu. As the plane began to taxi down the runway

---

34   Serious incidents are defined as events where there was no loss of life or serious injury or structural damage to a plane, but there was a significant risk of an accident having occurred.

there was a loud noise, which the pilot initially interpreted as a burst tyre. Take-off was immediately aborted but it was soon recognised that the noise had not been from a tyre but from an explosion in one of the engines, which led to a fuel tank bursting into flames. An immediate evacuation was ordered, but despite the heroic efforts of the cabin staff, not everyone could get out in time. Fifty-three passengers and two of the cabin crew died, nearly all from smoke inhalation, and a number of others sustained severe burns.

The crash investigators established that a major cause of the fatalities had been the difficulties in effecting an evacuation with the emergency exits becoming obstructed. A further aggravating factor was that the seat fabric was highly flammable and, once alight, emitted toxic fumes. On the recommendation of the AAIB, the Civil Aviation Authority (CAA) commissioned a research programme at the Cranfield Institute for Safety, Risk and Reliability[35] under a brilliant aeronautic psychologist, Professor Helen Muir, into how people evacuate from planes in a simulated emergency situation. They set up two full size aircraft fuselages and filmed and timed volunteers attempting to escape. Obviously, with an experiment they could not use real fire and smoke, so in order to artificially create an element of panic and chaos they offered financial incentives to the first people to get out, with a diminishing reward the longer people took.

The results paved the way to the reconfiguration of seating as we now know it, with wider spacing in the rows where the emergency exits are located, and care taken to ensure that

---

35 Generally called 'The Cranfield Institute' and now part of Cranfield University.

those in these rows do not have any mobility issues and know how to open the doors. In addition, the signage and floor level lighting, widening of bulkhead passageways and use of flame-retardant materials became standard in aircraft all over the world. These changes have undoubtedly saved countless lives.

Cranfield was subsequently commissioned to do additional research after the last fatal air disaster in the UK, at Kegworth in 1989, when a British Midland Boeing 737 hit a motorway embankment while attempting an emergency landing. Forty-seven of the 126 people on board died, but a remarkable number of those who survived were largely unscathed or had trivial injuries. Examination showed that most of those who died had failed to adopt the 'brace position' whereas those who survived unhurt had. Cranfield was able, using crash dummies and computer simulation, to reproduce these findings and to suggest modifications to the brace position.

Better systems of investigation have transformed aviation safety, but could they be adopted in healthcare? One influential doctor, Sir Liam Donaldson,[36] who from 1998 to 2010 held the position of Chief Medical Officer (CMO) for England, and who as such was the UK government's principal adviser on medical issues, certainly thought so. In 2001, a 17-year-old, Wayne Jowett, was the victim of a rare but recurring catastrophic adverse event in the course of treatment for leukaemia when he was given the drug vincristine by intrathecal injection (into

---

36 The role of Chief Medical Officer was established in 1855, and Donaldson was the 15th person to hold the position. The present incumbent (the 17th), Professor Chris Whitty, has, thanks to COVID-19, become a familiar face in the media, but the role is normally a very important but somewhat anonymous one.

the spinal fluid) rather than intravenously and died four weeks later. Donaldson immediately announced that the incident would be investigated by a highly experienced incident inspector, Professor Brian Toft. He had previously been involved in the investigation of the Ladbroke Grove rail crash and the *Marchioness* sinking on the River Thames in 1959 in which 51 people died when a pleasure boat twice collided with a barge. Professor Toft's investigation was to be conducted in the style of a rail or aircraft crash inquiry, to establish the facts and to learn lessons rather than to apportion blame.

Vincristine is a chemical that was discovered in the 1950s in the leaves of the rose periwinkle, *Catharanthus roseus*, a plant that had long been used in folk remedies. Investigation showed that it had a potent effect in suppressing the white blood count and this led to studies in the early 1960s which showed that it was remarkably effective in treating the commonest form of childhood cancer, acute lymphoblastic leukaemia, which had hitherto invariably been fatal. An early study from Great Ormond Street Hospital in London showed that intravenous injections of vincristine produced remission in virtually 100% of cases.

Unfortunately, vincristine does not cross the 'blood–brain barrier', the membrane that surrounds the central nervous system, and thus leukaemia was commonly found to relapse because of recurrence around the brain. Treatment regimens were therefore established to combine intravenous vincristine with injections of other cytotoxic drugs into the cerebrospinal fluid by means of a lumbar puncture, a needle passed into the spinal fluid in the lumbar region. Vincristine could not be used for this purpose because it was known to be highly toxic to nerve tissue. In fact, the first reported case of death following intrathecal injection of vincristine was reported in 1968, and nearly every case where the drug has been injected in this way has proved fatal. The very few survivors have been left with profound neurological disability. There is no effective treatment.

In the UK, at least a dozen cases of fatal vincristine toxicity from intrathecal injection had occurred before Wayne Jowett's. In 1997, a child had died at Great Ormond Street Hospital five days after the inadvertent intrathecal injection of the drug. The two junior doctors involved were charged with manslaughter, but were found not guilty at the Old Bailey after the Crown Prosecution Service (CPS) dropped charges. The CPS decided that the death was caused by a catalogue of 'chance events and failings' at the hospital, rather than gross negligence by the doctors. The judge accepted that a 'chapter of accidents and misunderstandings' at the hospital accounted for the child's death.

Professor Toft's investigation began almost immediately after Wayne Jowett's death. The sequence of events was as follows: Wayne Jowett was diagnosed with acute lymphoblastic leukaemia (ALL) in June 1999, and was treated by the haematology department at Queen's Medical Centre (QMC), Nottingham, one of 17 departments in the UK which treat this disorder. Wayne was treated using a UK Medical Research Council (MRC) trial protocol and by June 2000 was in remission, but was thereafter placed on a maintenance regime to prevent relapse. This required an injection each three months of intravenous vincristine and intrathecal cytosine (a cytotoxic drug which does not damage the nervous system), together with oral medication taken on a continuous basis. He was to be seen each month by the consultant haematologist, with a blood test at each visit.

According to the trial protocol, the intravenous and intrathecal injections were to be given on the same day but, as a safety measure, the department at QMC had agreed that their patients would have their injections on sequential days, the intravenous on the first and the intrathecal on the next. This had become standard procedure in the department.

Between June and December 2000, Wayne had missed two of his appointments and there were concerns with his compliance with his medication. Just before Christmas 2000 he requested that his next treatment be postponed until after Christmas and the New Year. An appointment was booked for 4th January 2001, but a note was not made in the ward diary for the drugs to be ordered in advance.

In the event, Wayne did not attend his appointment with the consultant on the morning of 4th January, and the ward staff were therefore not expecting him when he arrived in the afternoon, anticipating having his chemotherapy. As no patients had been scheduled for chemotherapy that afternoon, there were only two doctors on duty, both relatively junior. One was a senior house officer (SHO) who had recently joined the department on a four-month placement as part of his training in general medicine, but without any specialist knowledge and experience. The other was a specialist registrar (SpR) in haematology; that is, a qualified doctor training to be a haematologist, who had only joined the department two days earlier and who was supposed to be 'shadowing' for his first two weeks. He had previously worked in a training grade at another hospital, and had moved from Leicester Royal Infirmary (LRI) to QMC as part of his training programme.

Normally, drugs for patients having chemotherapy each week were ordered from the pharmacy on the preceding Thursday, but on the 4th January it had been noted that Wayne's medications had not been ordered. The consultant haematologist who was due to see him that morning wrote a prescription for cytosine IT (intrathecal) for the 4th January and vincristine IV (intravenous) for the 5th January. Normal procedure for the pharmacy would be for the two drugs to be sent back to the ward separately and on different days, but when Wayne arrived unexpectedly, a ward nurse rang the pharmacy asking that his medication should be sent to the ward urgently, and both drugs were sent together, in a single bag, and placed in the ward drug refrigerator. It was entirely contrary to normal practice for the two different drugs, intended for two different routes of administration, to be placed in a single bag and stored together in the drug refrigerator. To compound the risk, both drugs are colourless, and the syringes contain approximately the same volume.

The SHO, who had only once previously performed an intrathecal injection, was approached by a ward nurse who advised that Wayne required an intrathecal injection, and that she would ask the SpR to supervise. The SpR, in his previous hospital, had worked with a system where vincristine would never be present when intrathecal drugs were being administered, but had encountered two different drugs being given at the same time (cytosine and methotrexate).

I have described the scenario in some detail because it becomes easier to understand how this was an accident waiting to happen, and inevitably did. Both vincristine and cytosine were administered through the lumbar puncture needle, and Wayne Jowett died four weeks later.

Professor Toft in his conclusion reports, 'The evidence presented to this inquiry suggests that the adverse incident that led to Mr Jowett's death was not caused by one or even several human errors but by a far more complex amalgam of human, organisational, technical and social interactions'. He ends his report by stating, 'If we are looking back upon a decision which has been taken, as most decisions, in the absence of complete information, it is important that we should not assess the actions of decision-makers too harshly in the light of the knowledge which hindsight gives us'.

A coroner's inquest recorded a verdict of 'accidental death', but the police arrested both the SHO and the SpR on a charge of manslaughter. The charge against the SHO was subsequently dropped, but in September 2003, two-and-a-half years after Wayne Jowett's death, the SpR was sentenced to eight months' imprisonment. As he had already served 11 months in custody, he was immediately released, much to the disgust of the Jowett family. It would seem that, despite the CMO and Professor Toft's intentions, medicine had reverted to the old principle of the aviation industry in blaming the pilot and 'resuming flying as usual'.[37]

---

37   Sir Liam Donaldson's efforts were not entirely in vain. It is now standard for vincristine to be administered in a 50ml 'minibag', such a volume being almost impossible to give by the intrathecal route.

In fairness to Sir Liam Donaldson, he has continued to campaign for patient safety and had done so in the World Health Organization (WHO) for whom he had worked since leaving his role as CMO. Indeed, it was hearing an inspirational lecture that he gave in 2001 which stimulated my own interest in the subject.

Intrathecal administration of vincristine is not the only example of a type of medical safety issue known as 'wrong route drug administration', as illustrated in the tragic case of a young nurse called Mayra Cabrera.

Mayra was born in the Philippines and in 2002 came to the United Kingdom to work as a theatre nurse at the Great Western Hospital, Swindon. In May 2004, she was delivered of a baby son, Zac, in the maternity department of the hospital where she worked. She and her husband, Arnel, were overjoyed, and there is a photograph of a happy Mayra holding her newborn child. A few minutes later she had a cardiac arrest from which she could not be revived.

Whilst attempts were being made to resuscitate her, medical staff noticed that a drip which had been set up during her labour and which was supposed to be infusing saline solution into a vein had, in fact, been connected to a 500ml bag of Bupivacaine. This is a local anaesthetic used for epidural analgesia and which is potentially fatal when given intravenously. It was calculated that she had received an intravenous dose of 150ml, which would certainly have been sufficient to kill her.

Despite the pathologist's report, following a postmortem

examination that the cause of death had been the intravenous administration of Bupivacaine, the hospital advised Mr Cabrera that his wife's death had been due to natural causes. To add insult to injury, the Home Office advised him that, as he had only been allowed to come to the UK as his wife had had an 'essential worker' work permit, he must return to the Philippines.[38] In 2005, Mr Cabrera, through friends in the UK, instructed a rather dogged solicitor, Seamus Edney (a man not afraid of a David versus Goliath battle), and in due course the Great Western Hospital Trust admitted that the cause of death had been the erroneous administration of Bupivacaine in place of saline in the maternity department. A substantial out of court settlement was made in favour of Mayra's widowed husband and her son.

A coroner's inquest finally sat in 2008 and lasted four weeks. It established that there had been *two* previous deaths in the NHS from 'wrong route' administration of Bupivacaine, both of which antedated Mrs Cabrera's case. There had also been *three* previous non-fatal cases in the maternity department at Swindon. Although the hospital had established a policy that saline and Bupivacaine should never be stored together and that Bupivacaine should always be kept in a locked cupboard, these simple rules had not been followed.

After 17 hours of deliberation, the jury verdict gave a verdict of unlawful killing by gross negligence manslaughter by both the hospital Trust and of the midwife who had failed to check the drug. It was the first such verdict ever brought against a

---

38 In 2008, there was a last-minute change of heart by the Home Secretary, and Mr Cabrera was given leave to remain.

hospital Trust. The police passed the file to the CPS but, in the event, it was the Health and Safety Executive (HSE) that took matters further. In 2010, the Swindon and Marlborough NHS pleaded guilty to a charge brought by the HSE and were fined £75,000 with a further £25,000 in costs for breaches in health and safety legislation.

Richard Matthews QC, for the prosecution, said, 'Mayra Cabrera's death was caused by a drug error and the trust failed to undertake measures to stop that risk. As such, the trust's failure was a substantial cause of her death. Those breaches continued over a sustained period of time... The trust had prior knowledge that this was a tragedy waiting to happen'. The defence, true to form, attempted to deflect blame onto the individual midwife.

The judge, Mr Justice Clarke, said, 'No-one could be unmoved by this tragedy. No-one who knew what lay behind it could be untroubled at the systematic and individual fault which this inquiry revealed'.

No disciplinary action was ever brought by the hospital or the Nursing and Midwifery Council (NMC) against the midwife who had administered the Bupivacaine, and who had retired by the time of the inquest. Nor was any action brought against the hospital pharmacy staff, who would have ultimately been responsible for the safe storage of drugs. But the real tragedy was that a death occurred in circumstances which could have been avoided if the most elementary safety precautions had been taken, and a little boy was left to grow up without his mother. Once again, the NHS had failed to learn from its mistakes and, worryingly, little has been done to prevent a future repetition.

CHAPTER 4

Where There's a Will There's a Way

Local newspapers seem to be something of a dying industry, some 40% of them having ceased publication in recent years and many others are struggling. But Phil Coleman is an award-winning local journalist who still takes his professional responsibilities seriously. His official title is Chief Reporter for *The Westmorland Gazette*[39] and *The Carlisle News & Star* but in fact, these days, he is their only remaining full-time reporter. In October 2018, Phil found himself sitting in solitary splendour on the press benches in Carlisle Crown Court, listening to the trial of Dr Zholia Alemi, an NHS consultant psychiatrist who had worked as a doctor in the UK for 22 years, and who was charged with having forged the will of one of her elderly patients suffering from advanced dementia, with the intention on becoming the sole beneficiary of her estate, worth some £1.5 million.

After a trial lasting six days, Alemi was found guilty and sentenced to five years in prison. In sentencing her, Judge James Atkin said, 'This was despicable, cruel criminality

---

39 *The Westmorland Gazette* was founded in 1819; one of its early editors was Thomas de Quincey and contributors over the years have included William Wordsworth, Beatrix Potter and John Ruskin.

motivated by pure greed and you must be severely punished for it'. But something was twitching in Phil Coleman's journalistic antennae. As he said afterwards, 'It didn't seem likely that a crime of that magnitude would be a first offence'. His instinct was correct – Zholia Alemi had never been a doctor at all.

'Dr' Alemi was born in Iran, but had moved to New Zealand and enrolled at the University of Auckland to study medicine. But when Phil made phone calls to the university and to the Medical Council of New Zealand, they confirmed that she had never graduated and had therefore never qualified as a doctor. She had instead presented forged certificates to the General Medical Council (GMC) in Britain, the body that has the statutory duty to register medical practitioners and provide them a licence to practice. Her registration was recorded by the GMC as University of Auckland, 1982, BM, ChB.[40] Armed with registration from the GMC (no 4246372), Alemi was able to work as a doctor in the NHS for 22 years, but all along she was a fake, no more entitled to call herself a doctor than the hospital porter. For his journalistic scoop, Phil Coleman was, in 2019, nominated for the highly prestigious *Private Eye* Paul Foot Award[41] for campaigning and investigative journalism, and was one of the runners-up.

Zholia Alemi had worked for most of those 22 years as a 'consultant psychiatrist' in various parts of the UK, including Plymouth, Norfolk and Suffolk, South Yorkshire and Humberside, Cumbria, and for six health boards in Scotland,

---

40 Bachelor of Medicine, Bachelor of Surgery.

41 The award was established in memory of the *Private Eye* and *The Guardian* journalist, Paul Foot, who died in 2004.

from Ayrshire and Arran in the West, to Dundee on the East, the Borders in the South and Inverness in the Highlands. She also attended Mental Health Tribunals in Scotland over a five-year period, when the continued hospitalisation of psychiatric patients admitted under section was determined, sitting in some 85 cases. All of these various employers would have relied on the GMC's Medical Register to confirm her status as a qualified doctor, as would any patients or relatives who wished to check her credentials.

In August 2020, Alemi was further charged by the police with eight counts of fraud by false representation and other matters, relating to having misrepresented herself to NHS employers. At the time of writing, she is yet to come to trial on these additional charges.

As a consultant psychiatrist, she would have been involved in treating vulnerable patients with severe mental health problems, including authorising their compulsory detention or release into the community and the prescribing of highly potent psychoactive drugs and electroconvulsive therapy (ECT), all without any medical qualifications. The GMC, whose primary purpose is to 'protect, promote and maintain the health and safety of the public', promptly issued an apology 'for any risk arising to patients' but what damage she may have done will probably never be known. Several of her past employers have announced that they will conduct reviews of patients treated under her care, but how feasible this will be is difficult to know; many will have died, or have moved away, or may have continuing mental health issues that will make this sort of investigation impossible.

It was the GMC's claim that Alemi was able to obtain registration through a loophole in their registration system. Until 1993, doctors who had qualified in medicine in Commonwealth countries (including New Zealand) were exempt from taking the Professional and Linguistic Assessments Board (PLAB) test, which those from other countries had to take when seeking to register in the UK. But this seems to miss the point in that, even if the PLAB test *had* applied to Alemi, she would have had to produce her exam certificates and these would have been forgeries. In fact, after Phil Coleman had unmasked her as a fraud, the GMC contacted over 3,000 UK doctors who had qualified in Commonwealth countries before 1993 and arranged for their qualifications to be re-checked.

But should the GMC have been so blind to the possibility of fake doctors? Some 20 years ago I organised a Saturday morning teaching session on dermatology for the GPs in my area, and thought it would be a nice touch if I gave them each a certificate of attendance. I am not terribly skilled when it comes to computers, and was even less so then, but I was rather pleased with my handywork when, a few days before the meeting, I produced a splendid A4 size certificate to present to each of the attendees. But as I looked at it, a rather worrying thought came to me; if someone with my very limited computer skills and artistic ability could make a certificate, how easy would it be for someone to make one for the purposes of deception?

The NHS has, from the outset, welcomed doctors from overseas, and the health service would never have functioned without them. In the early years, they came predominantly from the Indian subcontinent, South Africa, Australia and New Zealand, so the GMC would no doubt have been familiar with the medical schools and universities in those countries and the different types of documentation they provided. But from the 1990s onwards, doctors were coming to the UK from an enlarging European Union (EU) and from the now-liberated countries of the old communist bloc. The question that bothered me was: how would the GMC know how to determine the authenticity of a medical degree certificate presented by a would-be doctor from a country with which they weren't particularly familiar?

I had no specific concerns in mind and, indeed, over the years I have had excellent colleagues from almost every corner of the globe, but I phoned the GMC and had a long and slightly puzzling conversation with them. I asked how they knew whether a certificate from abroad was genuine. Did they, for example, keep an album of genuine certificates from different countries? And, furthermore, what would happen if someone came from a country or from a medical school from which no doctor had ever previously registered? I remember giving them a hypothetical example of a doctor from Outer Mongolia presenting an impressive certificate from the University of Ulan Bator. I cannot say that I was reassured by their answers. They seemed genuinely perplexed by the idea that a doctor would be capable of telling a lie. I wasn't totally convinced, but I didn't think that it was for me to pursue the matter.

I was not the only person who had these concerns. In 1996, a researcher at the University of Bath, Joanne Hartland, published a paper in the magazine *Health Service Journal (HSJ)* identifying some 30 instances of fake doctors working in the

NHS.[42] In 2002, an article appeared in the *British Medical Journal (The BMJ)*[43] reporting that the Indian Medical Council, India's equivalent of the GMC (and now called the National Medical Commission [NMC]), was no longer going to allow Indian subjects who had obtained medical diplomas in Russia or the countries of the former Soviet Union[44] to practice medicine because some 40-50% of their diplomas were believed to have been fakes. More recently, the Pakistan Medical and Dental Council has followed suit with respect to degrees issued both in Russia and China.

By 2013, the Russian authorities were so concerned about the scale of fake degree certificates and diplomas, not only in medicine but also in law, science and engineering, that it set up a new government body to attempt to regulate matters, the Federal Service for Supervision in Education and Science. The first page of the website carries the slogan '**STOP CORRUPTION**' and the telephone number of its anti-corruption hotline is prominently displayed.[45]

In 2015, 36-year-old Levon Mkhitarian, originally from Georgia, was sentenced to six years in prison at Canterbury Crown Court, after being found guilty of having fraudulently worked as a doctor for two years using fake documentation at William Harvey Hospital, Ashford, Kent. He had originally

---

42 Masquerade: tracking the bogus doctors, *J Hartland Health Service Journal* 1996, vol 106:26–29.

43 S Kumar. Medical degrees from former Soviet countries are under question. *British Medical Journal* 2002, vol 325(7358):238.

44 This had at the time been a popular route into a medical career for Indians who had failed to secure a place at an Indian medical school.

45 +7 (495) 608-7485, in case you feel the need to call it.

come to the UK in 2007 on a student visa and had been granted provisional registration by the GMC; this had been withdrawn when they were not satisfied with his ability to practice safely, prompting Mkhitarian into a life of deceit.

And in 2017, BBC TV showed a fictional drama, with Jodie Whittaker in the lead role, about a fake doctor. The series was written by a doctor, Dan Sefton, who admitted in an interview with BBC News that he had once worked with a doctor who subsequently turned out not to be a doctor at all.

Notwithstanding these warnings, when Zholia Alemi's fake qualifications came to light, the GMC's Director admitted in a letter to me that the GMC did not indeed have the technical expertise to validate foreign certificates and that they paid a private company in the USA, the Educational Commission for Foreign Medical Graduates (ECFMG), based in Pennsylvania, to do this for them.

As touched upon earlier, it is not only in medicine that fraudulent qualifications can lead to catastrophe. In May 2020, a Pakistan International Airlines (PIA) flight from Lahore to Karachi crashed on attempting to land, having overshot the runway and careering into a nearby housing estate. All but two of those on board, and several people on the ground, were killed. There was nothing particularly unusual about a PIA plane crashing for the airline has had a catastrophic safety record in recent years; however, what was chilling was that neither of the pilots were qualified. A government investigation revealed that a staggering 150 of the pilots flying for PIA, about a third of the total, had fake pilots' licences or had paid someone else to take their exams for them. Even more concerning was the fact that the problem had been under investigation since 2018.

Zholia Alemi's case was certainly a wake up call for the GMC, and possibly for other professional regulatory bodies, but it certainly was not the first case where the GMC was not as vigilant as it might have been in performing its duty in protecting the public.

By a rather peculiar coincidence, it had been an attempt to forge a will that had led to the unmasking of the GP, Dr Harold Shipman, as a mass murderer. On 24th June 1998, the last of Shipman's victims, 81-year-old Kathleen Grundy, a former mayoress of Hyde and a sprightly lady for her age, was found dead at her home, just a few hours after Dr Shipman had visited her, ostensibly to take a blood sample. Shipman signed a death certificate giving, as the cause of death, 'old age'.

On the same day, a letter arrived at Mrs Grundy's solicitor containing a new will, and a covering letter. The will excluded Mrs Grundy's children and left the whole estate, worth £368,000 to Shipman. The will read, 'I give all my estate, money and house to my doctor. My family are not in need and I want to reward him for all the care he has given to me and the people of Hyde'. The accompanying letter, which had clearly been prepared on the same typewriter, subsequently shown to be a *Brother* portable typewriter owned by Shipman, stated:

'Dear Sir, I enclose a copy of my will, I wish Dr Shipman to benefit by having my estate but if he dies or cannot accept it then my estate goes to my daughter. I would like you to be the executor of the will. I intend to make an appointment to discuss this and my will in the near future.'

The solicitor, Brian Burgess, was sufficiently concerned to contact Mrs Grundy's daughter, Angela Woodruff, herself a lawyer who had previously supervised all her mother's financial affairs and who promptly recognised that the signature was not her mother's. At Burgess' suggestion, Mrs Woodruff contacted the police.

Earlier in the year, in March 1998, the proprietor of a local funeral directors, Frank Massey and Sons, approached another local general practice, concerned about the high death rate among Dr Shipman's patients. The GPs themselves had noticed the unusually large number of cremation forms that they were being asked to countersign relating to his patients. A cremation form has to be signed by two doctors, and Dr Shipman was in single-handed practice. One of the GPs, Dr Linda Reynolds, had noted that an unusual number of patients seemed to have died in the middle of the afternoon, fully clothed and often midway through a cup of tea or cigarette. Also, unusually, the deaths seemed to have occurred during or shortly after a visit from Shipman. An approach was made to the coroner for South Manchester, John Pollard, who in turn contacted the police. The police delegated the matter to two rather junior detectives, who appeared not to have shown much interest and, indeed, had not troubled to interview Shipman or any of the relatives of the deceased, and the matter was subsequently closed the next month. Nor had the police ever actually troubled to check Shipman's record, and so were unaware that he had a criminal record for drugs offences from 1976.

However, Mrs Woodruff's new approach finally set alarm bells ringing. Mrs Grundy's body was exhumed from Hyde Cemetery at 4 am on 1st August, the first exhumation *ever* conducted by the Greater Manchester Police (GMP). A detailed postmortem examination was conducted, which revealed high levels of diamorphine (medical grade heroin), in her system. When challenged, Shipman claimed, somewhat improbably, that Mrs Grundy was a drug addict and showed them her medical records to this effect on his practice computer. However, GP computers track the dates on which entries are made and will log retrospective changes, so it was simple to demonstrate that he had changed the records after the event. Finding Shipman's fingerprints on Mrs Grundy's will completed the trail of evidence.

Shipman was arrested on 7th September 1998 and, after a review of further cases, he appeared at Preston Crown Court the following month charged with 15 counts of murder, though ultimately his activities are believed to have been the cause of death of some 250 of his patients. In every case there had been an injection of diamorphine on doubtful medical grounds shortly before death and a retrospective change in the case records to indicate, falsely, that the subject had been in poor health. In the great majority of cases, the body had been cremated, eliminating the possibility of forensic evidence. Curiously, Mrs Grundy's was the only case where Shipman stood to profit from a will; Shipman never offered any explanation for his activities.

On 31st January 2000, after a trial that had lasted nearly four months, and after six days of deliberation, the jury found Shipman guilty of all 15 counts of murder[46] and one of

---

46 The 15 were, in addition to Mrs Grundy, Marie West, Irene Turner, Lizzie Adams, Jean Lilley, Ivy Lomas, Muriel Grimshaw, Marie Quinn, Kathleen Wagstaff, Bianka Pomfret, Norah Nuttall, Pamela Hillier, Maureen Ward, Winifred Mellor and Joan Melia.

forgery. He was sentenced to life imprisonment for each of the murders, with a recommendation that he should never be released and a further four years on the forgery charge. On 11th February, the GMC formally erased Shipman's name from the Medical Register. Shipman never acknowledged his crimes and disputed the scientific evidence. On 13th January 2004, Shipman was found dead in his cell at Wakefield Prison, having hanged himself using his bed sheets, which were tied to the bars on the window.

Inevitably, Shipman's conviction caused public consternation. Just how could an apparently diligent and well-liked GP practising in a small nondescript market town seven miles from Manchester really be the worst mass murderer in British legal history?[47] Particular focus was directed to the GMC, the organisation which had the statutory duty to licence and regulate doctors. How could they possibly have allowed a doctor to have acted in this way?

The day after Shipman's conviction, the Secretary of State for Health and Social Care, Alan Milburn, announced that there would be an independent inquiry, to be held in private, but with its findings made public. The inquiry began under Lord Laming of Tewin, a former social worker, but there was uproar

---

47 As far as I can establish, no-one in the press commented on the fact that Hyde had also been where Ian Brady and Myra Hindley, the 'Moors Murderers', had lived, and where they were arrested. Brady and Hindley murdered five children between 1963 and 1965. The body of one of them, Keith Bennett, has never been discovered.

Hyde is also where Dale Cregan was arrested in 2012. He was convicted of murdering two police officers, Fiona Bone and Nicola Hughes, and two others; his crime was unique – the first conviction in the United Kingdom where a hand grenade was the murder weapon.

in the media and anger among the relatives of the deceased and, after successful legal action, a formal public inquiry was established under Dame Janet Smith, the High Court Judge, who had formerly been a barrister specialising in personal injury and medical negligence cases, and who had previously conducted an inquiry into the abuse of children with autism in a care home. Dame Janet's report, generally called *The Shipman Inquiry*, was published in six parts, the final one appearing in 2006.

The fifth part of Dame Janet Smith's report focused on the deficiencies of the GMC in having failed to protect the public. Her criticisms were scathing. 'Having examined the evidence, I have been driven to the conclusion that the GMC has not, in the past, succeeded in its primary purpose of protecting patients', Dame Janet said. Even the GMC itself, in giving evidence, admitted that it had failed to meet the reasonable expectations of patients and the public.

True to form, the GMC decided that the best defence was to blame other people. Shipman had been in single-handed General Practice, but six GPs from neighbouring surgeries, Drs Peter Bennett, Rajesh Patel, Jeremy Dirckze, Stephen Farrar, Alastair MacGillivray and Susan Booth were summoned to appear before a GMC Fitness to Practice Panel, charged with serious professional misconduct, by virtual of having countersigned cremation forms relating to some of Shipman's patients. These hearings, which have the power to erase a doctor's name from the Medical Register (and thereby end their career), have long been regarded with considerable suspicion by doctors because the GMC acted as investigator, judge and jury and so they are effectively a 'kangaroo court'.

Dame Janet Smith's report described the process as not being fit for purpose, and called for its radical reform.[48]

Even by the standards of the GMC, the case against the six doctors was plainly absurd and was ultimately abandoned. The first legal cremation in Britain took place in Woking, Surrey, in 1885, the culmination of a long campaign led by the eminent surgeon, Sir Henry Thompson,[49] although it was not until the Cremation Act 1902 that its legal basis was fully established.

One obvious and entirely reasonable public anxiety was that, once a body had been cremated, there would be no possibility of further examination if doubt were later cast about the cause of death. It had, indeed, been the good fortune of the police that Shipman's last victim, Mrs Grundy, had been buried, as it had proved possible to exhume her body and take samples for measurement of diamorphine, something that had not been possible in most of the other deaths where the deceased had been cremated. The Cremation Act requires two doctors to each complete a Cremation Certificate. The first of these would normally be the GP if the patient had died in the

---

48 In recent years, the system has changed so that investigations are conducted by the GMC and the hearings by a separate body, the Medical Practitioners Tribunal Service (MPTS) but, in reality, the two work hand in glove. I have never had to appear before them but I have, on a number of occasions, been paid by the GMC to act as an expert advisor in cases being investigated and have found them very challenging taskmasters. In one case, I recall being asked to give my opinion on documents so heavily redacted that they were simply incomprehensible, and yet a senior doctor's entire professional life was at stake. There have been an alarming number of cases where entirely innocent doctors have found the whole process so oppressive that they have committed suicide.

49 Thompson was a member of Queen Victoria's medical household. He was an authority on the treatment of bladder stones, and operated on both King Leopold of Belgium and the exiled Emperor Napoleon III.

community, or a hospital doctor if they had died in hospital. If it was the former, they would have to have been familiar with the patient before their death and to be in a position to identify the medical cause of death. If the death was sudden or unexplained, they would not be able to sign the form without the permission of the coroner. The signatory has to confirm that there is no evidence that the death was violent or unnatural.

A second confirmatory form has to be signed by another doctor unconnected with the care of the patient, and if a GP had signed the first form, the second signatory would have to be from a different practice.[50] They will have inspected the body, spoken with the GP who had cared for the patient, and signed that '...*to the best of my knowledge and belief and that I know of no reasonable cause to suspect that the deceased died either a violent or unnatural death or a sudden death of which the cause is unknown or in a place or circumstance which requires an inquest in pursuance of any Act.*' There is then a final check whereby both certificates are carefully reviewed by the medical referee at the crematorium.[51]

The idea that the GPs who had countersigned Shipman's Cremation Certificates might have detected that he was a mass murder was entirely fanciful. It was not their role, nor were they trained, to perform a postmortem examination or to take blood samples for poisons. A GP might decline to countersign

---

50 The requirement for the second Confirmatory Cremation Certificate was suspended in April 2020 as part of the coronavirus regulations.

51 The exact wording has changed slightly over the years, and the arrangements are slightly different in Scotland, but the principles of two independent signatories has remained. The certificates cannot be signed if either party is uncertain as to the medical cause of death or if there is any suspicion of foul play, nor if either has any pecuniary interest in the death.

the form if the Cause of Death did not match the history given, or if inspection of the body revealed unexplained injuries such as gunshot or stab wounds or signs of strangulation, or in the unlikely event of there being the 'burnt almond' smell encountered in cyanide poisoning, but there would have been nothing in the evidence presented to them in any of Shipman's cases which would have aroused the suspicions even of Miss Marple or Hercule Poirot. And of course, by March 1998 when the numbers of cases were noted to be out of order, they had notified the coroner, and through him the police, but little had been done.

The GMC had, however, missed a much earlier opportunity to bring Shipman's murderous behaviour to a halt. In 1963, when Shipman was 17, his mother, who was only 43, was diagnosed with an advanced form of lung cancer, and was treated at home by the GP, who used to visit daily to give injections of an opiate painkiller. Shipman was said to have been close to his mother and seems at this time to have developed an unnatural and abiding fascination with these potent drugs. He qualified in medicine at Leeds University Medical School and, after junior hospital positions in Pontefract, in 1974 he secured a position at the Albert Ormerod Medical Centre in Todmorden, on the Yorkshire-Lancashire border. The other GPs in the practice found him diligent and hard working, and one of the additional duties he volunteered to take on was the disposal of a quantity of Controlled Drugs[52] that were out of date, and to take responsibility for ordering new supplies. By February 1975,

---

52   Controlled Drugs are drugs specified by the Misuse of Drugs Act, which are potentially addictive and for which special controls on storage, supply and prescription apply; they include morphine, pethidine and diamorphine (heroin).

the Home Office Drugs Inspectorate and the West Yorkshire Police drug squad became aware that Shipman was ordering unusually large quantities of pethidine from local pharmacies. Enquiries were made and they were satisfied that Shipman was not a drug addict. In June 1975, a pharmaceutical supplier noted the very large quantities of pethidine being supplied to the Boots branch at Todmorden, ordered by Dr Shipman, who was interviewed by the Drugs Inspectorate and the police. It was noted that the surgery records relating to Controlled Drugs were inadequate. The Drugs Inspectorate made a further visit in August 1975 and arranged to return in a further six months.

Meanwhile, Shipman had started experiencing health problems, including blackouts. Initially, a diagnosis of epilepsy was made but, in September 1975, his partners at the practice confronted him and he admitted he had been obtaining large quantities of pethidine for his personal use. He was immediately admitted to the local hospital and then to The Retreat, a psychiatric hospital near York. The psychiatrists notified the Home Office that Shipman should be registered as a drug addict. In November 1975, Shipman was interviewed by the police at The Retreat, and made a detailed statement which included the words 'I have no future intention to return to General Practice or work in a situation where I could obtain supplies of pethidine'. He was discharged from hospital at the end of 1975 with the advice that he should stay under psychiatric supervision for several years.

On 13th February 1976, Shipman appeared at the Halifax Magistrates' Court, where he pleaded guilty to eight specimen charges: three offences of obtaining ten ampoules of 100mg pethidine by deception, three of unlawfully possessing pethidine and two of forging a prescription. He asked for 74 further offences to be taken into consideration. Shipman was fined £75 on each charge, £600 in all, and ordered to pay compensation of £58.78 to the local NHS Family Practitioners Committee.

As is routine when any doctor receives a criminal conviction, the GMC was notified. It was, at that time, its procedure for Shipman's case to be considered by the GMC's 'Penal Cases Committee', which met in April 1976. Detective Sergeant George McKeating, who had arrested Shipman and taken his statement in The Retreat, was called to the committee, but was astonished to find that he was never called to give evidence. Clearly, the GMC had made up its mind and was not going to let facts get in the way. In their view, Shipman was a chastened man and was not a risk to patients. The GMC advised the Home Office of their decision. The Home Office had the right to prevent Shipman from having access to or prescribing Controlled Drugs, but were reassured the GMC decided to put no restrictions on him. The GMC did, however, send him a pamphlet on the hazards of drug misuse, so no doubt they felt that this fulfilled their duty of protecting the public.

Even more extraordinarily, the GMC made no enquiry at all as to whether Shipman might have been harming patients. It was only after Shipman's conviction in 2000 that relatives of his Todmorden patients started coming forward expressing their concerns, and it became apparent that at least 15 had died under his care in suspicious circumstances. When this information emerged from *The Shipman Inquiry*, questions began emerging as to what had happened when he was a junior hospital doctor in Pontefract from 1970 to 1974. Investigation of events 30 years previously was necessarily challenging but it seems almost certain that it was then that his killing spree had begun.

Clearly, if the GMC had not been asleep, at the very least, Shipman's work after 1976 would have been closely monitored, his prescribing of Controlled Drugs restricted, and probably his working as a single-handed GP prevented; all these restrictions would have been entirely within the GMC's remit. Rather than bringing entirely bogus disciplinary action against the six GPs for countersigning cremation forms, the GMC might have properly reflected on its own inertia and the subsequent mass murders in Hyde.

One further issue that was never considered by either the GMC or *The Shipman Inquiry* was whether anyone had ever reviewed how Harold Shipman had even managed to become a doctor at all. The seeds of his early fascination with injecting drugs were no doubt sown watching his mother's final illness while he was an impressionable teenager. Could lessons have been learned for the future about assessing the psychological suitability of medical students for a career in the profession?

In the aftermath of the Shipman case, and before Dame Janet Smith had completed her inquiry, the GMC announced that they would be introducing a new mandatory system of checking on the performance of doctors, through a process of appraisal and revalidation. In fact, the idea of appraisal and revalidation for doctors had earlier been proposed by Professor Kennedy's 2001 inquiry into the scandal of paediatric cardiac surgery at Bristol between 1984 and 1995,[53] but nothing had actually happened. Under the GMC's new plan, each doctor would have a 'Responsible Officer'[54] and would undergo an annual 'appraisal' of their work. Every five years, they would undergo 'revalidation', when their licence to practice as a doctor would be renewed by the GMC on the basis of a recommendation by the Responsible Officer. A condition of revalidation would be the successful completion of annual appraisal in each of the preceding five years.

Dame Janet Smith gave the GMC's plans a half-hearted welcome, indicating that they were a start, but almost certainly would not have weeded out Dr Shipman. The annual appraisal is a burdensome process for doctors. You are required to get voluminous documentation and enter it into a complex database. Every article in a medical journal that you have read and every lecture you have attended in the preceding year must be recorded, along with your detailed account of what you learned. Every letter of complaint, however seemingly irrelevant ('the hospital car park was full') must be recorded, along with your comments. Every letter of thanks must also be included, but must first be defaced by obliterating the name of the grateful patient. Evidence of attendance at 'Mandatory Training' must be faithfully recorded, even though much of it bears no connection with how good or safe a doctor you are.[55]

---

53   See Chapter 8: 'The Heart of the Matter'.

54   In the case of hospital doctors, including consultants, the Responsible Officer would normally be the Medical Director of their hospital. In the case of a GP it would normally be a senior doctor from another practice.

55   At my last appraisal I had to provide evidence that I was up to date on Fire Safety, Manual Handling and Lifting, Information Governance, and Equality and Diversity Awareness; all important topics, but hardly relevant if the object is to ensure that I am not another mass murderer.

Evidence of your probity must be provided. An 'audit' of how you have performed against national targets must also be included.

When all this has been done, you must then have a formal meeting with your appraiser, usually a senior doctor from another department, or, in the case of general practice, from another practice. The meetings are invariably stressful and, although they can be constructive, can sometimes have the feel of a latter-day Spanish Inquisition. The whole process is challenging, and I know of a number of doctors for whom the appraisal process has been the trigger for early retirement. It is also time-consuming. Assembling and recording the documentation can rarely be completed in less than 50 hours each year, time that could otherwise be spent looking after patients.[56] Harold Shipman would almost certainly have breezed through the process; he was well liked by patients, well organised, an early advocate of computers and of audit in general practice and was also good at brushing off difficult questions.

Amazingly, having established a system for revalidating doctors, the person who the GMC appointed to run their revalidation programme, Lindsey Westwood, had no previous experience in healthcare and had previously worked as an appeals manager at the Traffic Penalty Tribunal. As a senior GP, Dr Vernon Coleman, wrote 'the person the GMC has put

---

56　For a GP's perspective on appraisal and revalidation, I commend an excellent article in *The Spectator* by GP Dr Vernon Coleman; a flavour of his views is suggested by the title 'Meet the Bloated Useless General Medical Council'.
　　The article may be found on the Internet: https://www.spectator.co.uk/article/meet-the-bloated-useless-general-medical-council.

in charge of checking the fitness to practise of every doctor in Britain was recently checking parking tickets for a living.'

Whilst Harold Shipman would almost certainly have eluded the GMC's appraisal and revalidation system, the fake doctor, Zholia Alemi, would and should have been stopped in her tracks if the system actually worked. She would have had to have gone through at least ten annual appraisals from the time that the system began, to when she was finally unmasked, plus two revalidation cycles. One obvious point that any appraisal should have covered was why she was moving from job to job with such regularity. Consultants are entitled to move, and many do, sometimes for family reasons, sometimes for professional ones but moving ten times, and from one end of the country to the other was very odd behaviour of a type that should have provoked enquiry.

Another even more serious matter was that Alemi had been reported to the GMC on at least nine occasions, and had to face a disciplinary panel of the GMC twice. On one occasion she was given a warning by the GMC for having failed to notify them of a criminal conviction (of careless driving), something which all doctors are bound to do. Doctors do, of course, have complaints made about them, but to have had nine complaints to the GMC and two disciplinary hearings in 22 years would have been so far out of the normal experience as to make serious investigation mandatory. It is certainly something that should have been considered in some detail during the annual appraisal process.

Even more remarkably, at one stage, notwithstanding all this, Alemi was actually considered for appointment as a

Responsible Officer at one of the hospitals where she worked; someone with entirely fake qualifications could have been judging whether other doctors could continue in practice. How she achieved this position is unexplained. It does seem extraordinary with her very odd pattern of employment, and the frequency of complaints about her being made to the GMC, that no-one there had applied the same degree of natural curiosity as Phil Coleman of *The Carlisle News & Star*.

In 2020, in the wake of the COVID-19 epidemic, appraisal and revalidation have been suspended. There is no evidence to date to indicate that, freed of this oppressive and inefficient regulatory burden, doctors have run amok.

CHAPTER 5

The Trial of the Century

In March 1957, Dr John Bodkin Adams, a GP from Eastbourne, stood in the dock of the Central Criminal Court (popularly called the 'Old Bailey' from the name of the road in which it stands), charged with murder. The case had created a sensation and was the front-page story in newspapers around the world. It was called, with some justification, 'the trial of the century'.[57] No British doctor had ever stood trial for the murder of a patient and, if convicted, he would be sentenced to hang. And just as in the cases of Harold Shipman and Zholia Alemi (discussed in Chapter 4), it was a will that brought him to attention, although in Bodkin Adams' case the wills weren't forged and he had received legacies from many dozens of his grateful patients.

Bodkin Adams was born in rural Ulster in 1899, raised in humble circumstances, and qualified in medicine from Queen's University of Belfast in 1921. His fellow pupils regarded him as 'a hardworking plodder'. The following year he moved to Eastbourne as a junior partner in a practice. At the time it was

---

57   There are many books about the case, but I recommend 'The Strange Case of Dr Bodkin Adams' written by a retired Eastbourne pathologist, Dr John Surtees. I am also grateful to my friend, Dr Keith Liddell, formerly Consultant Dermatologist at Eastbourne District General Hospital, who knew Bodkin Adams and gave me background information about the case.

a fashionable and wealthy town. Its sunny climate made it a popular place for elderly couples to retire and, inevitably, that meant that there were plenty of frail, lonely widows with time on their hands.

Medical practice was very different in those days. There were few effective treatments, and often the most that a GP could offer was a sympathetic ear and a kindly word and, in this, Bodkin Adams excelled. He was a rather rotund, jovial and talkative individual, and was happy to make himself available at all hours of day and night regardless of whether the patient was rich or poor. In the case of the latter, he often made no charge. In addition, he was a superb marksman, close to Olympic standard at clay pigeon shooting, which made him popular with the local aristocracy who were pleased to invite him to their shoots.

In 1935, an elderly widowed patient, Mrs Matilda Whitton, died, leaving her doctor, Dr Bodkin Adams, £7000 in her will. It was an enormous sum at the time; five years earlier he had bought a substantial house in one of the best streets in the town for £3000. The other local GPs, who had mostly come to Eastbourne from the smart London medical schools such as Guy's and St Thomas', were a rather snobbish bunch and had already come to resent his popularity with patients. Mrs Whitton's legacy certainly didn't improve his standing with his professional colleagues.

In those days it was also quite common for GPs to undertake sessions at the local hospital, and Bodkin Adams used to spend a couple of afternoons each week giving anaesthetics for surgical patients. Anaesthesia was far less complicated in that era, and Bodkin Adams was quite proficient at it having studied in his spare time for a Diploma in Anaesthesia. It was quite a hazardous undertaking, and it was easy for the person administering the anaesthetic gases to be overexposed to them as there were not the enclosed breathing systems which are standard nowadays. Whereas in the Shipman and Alemi cases the GMC may have been criticized for being 'asleep on the job', there were times when Bodkin Adams was literally so. One of the local surgeons recalls remarking as he completed an operation, 'Well, Bodkin, the patient's awake, isn't it time you woke up too?' His tendency to nod off wasn't assisted by the nurses plying him with cream cakes as he sat at the anaesthetic machine.

Whilst it wasn't totally out of the ordinary for GPs to be left money by patients, the frequency with which Bodkin Adams was a beneficiary and the size of the bequests continued to generate gossip, especially in a small town where the doctors, solicitors and bank managers all knew each other. In all, he was believed to have received bequests in some 134 patients' wills, and the total sums of money involved were very substantial. By the early 1950s he was said to have been the richest doctor in England, though whether that was true or not is hard to prove. He certainly had all the trappings of wealth, with a chauffeur-driven Rolls-Royce car and a pair of handmade Purdey shotguns which he took on his grouse shooting holidays. There was endless muttering about the frequency with which his patients wrote a will with him as a beneficiary and then soon afterwards died, often after an injection of morphine. However, this was essentially rumour and innuendo rather than solid fact.

One of his patients, Edith Morrell, was a wealthy and

rather unpleasant lady from Cheshire. She had had a stroke and suffered from arthritis, problems which did not improve her temperament. She had proven to be so difficult with her relatives that they packed her off to a nursing home in Eastbourne, and then, when she complained about that, to a private house where a bevy of nurses cared for her. Bodkin Adams looked after her as a private patient, and allowed himself to be at her beck and call at all hours of day and night. Mrs Morrell was in the habit of changing her will with remarkable frequency. Bodkin Adams went away for a few days' holiday in September 1950, and as soon as she realised that he had gone away she wrote a codicil to her will, cutting him out of it. He rushed back from his holiday and, by early October, his status as a beneficiary had been re-established.

For the two years or so that Mrs Morrell had been under Bodkin Adams' care, he had been giving her regular injections of diamorphine (heroin) to which it is almost certain that she had become addicted. He always insisted that the nurses leave the room when he gave her injections, and his record keeping was minimal, so exactly what was being given was unknown. Edith Morrell died on 13th November 1950 without any further changes to her will. Bodkin Adams signed her Cremation Certificate, and to the question, 'Do you have any pecuniary interest in the death?' had written, 'Not as far as I am aware'. In fact, he was to receive a chest of antique silverware and a Rolls-Royce Silver Ghost car.

Rumours of excessive prescribing of opiate drugs, wills and deaths continued until 1956. Gertrude 'Bobbie' Tomlinson was a rather vivacious but highly-strung lady of 48. She had been widowed some years before and, in 1953, Bodkin Adams introduced her to another of his wealthy patients, Jack Hullett, who himself was a widower. A whirlwind romance and marriage followed, and all was well until March 1956 when he suddenly died, a few months after an operation for cancer. He left Bodkin Adams £500 in his will.

Bobbie Hullett, as she now was, was distraught, and suffered a nervous breakdown. She frequently expressed a wish to die. Bodkin Adams did not seek any assistance from a psychiatrist, but treated her with phenobarbitone, a highly addictive and potentially toxic barbiturate and a prescription drug which was widely abused at the time.

On 18th July 1956, Bodkin Adams took a cheque for £1000 signed by Bobbie Hullett to the bank, asking for it to be cleared urgently, explaining to the clerk that 'This lady is not long for this world'. The following afternoon she was found deeply unconscious at home. Her maid called Bodkin Adams, who was unavailable, but arranged for another GP, Dr Harris, to visit. Bodkin Adams had failed to advise Dr Harris that Mrs Hullett had expressed suicidal ideas, nor that she was on barbiturates, so he had no reason to suspect a possible barbiturate overdose. Dr Harris, suspecting that she might have had a cerebral haemorrhage or possibly meningitis, considered that she ought to be admitted to hospital, but Bodkin Adams, when he became available, refused to allow this.

Mrs Hullett remained unconscious and, in the early hours of the next day, Bodkin Adams telephoned the coroner, asking his advice as to how to arrange a private postmortem. The coroner, Dr Sommerville, asked him when the patient had died, to which he received the startling reply, 'Oh, she isn't dead yet'.

The coroner, who had been woken from his sleep by the call, promptly slammed down the receiver.

Bobbie Hullett died in the early hours of 21st July. The cause of death was given by Bodkin Adams as 'cerebral haemorrhage'. Under the terms of her will, written only a few days before her death, he received yet another Rolls-Royce.

The circumstances were so extraordinary that the coroner arranged for a postmortem to be conducted by a Home Office pathologist, Professor Francis Camps. Tissue tests confirmed that Mrs Hullett had twice the fatal level of barbiturate in her system. The Chief Constable of the Eastbourne Constabulary[58] decided to call in Scotland Yard for the first time in its history.

As part of the investigation, Professor Camps reviewed the death certificates of all of Bodkin Adams' patients who had died, and discovered that an alarmingly high proportion had received injections of opiates (morphine or diamorphine) or barbiturates shortly before death. Some 164 cases were considered worthy of further investigation, and the possibility of a murder charge was considered in five, including both Edith Morrell and Bobbie Hullett. The police believed that there were 14 cases in which patients who had recently made Bodkin Adams a beneficiary of their will had died shortly afterwards, having been given an injection by him. Under questioning about Mrs Morrell, Bodkin Adams famously replied, 'Easing the passing of a dying patient is not all that wicked. She wanted to die; that cannot be murder.'

---

58 Eastbourne had its own police force at the time.

In such a high profile case, the final decision on bringing a prosecution is made by the Attorney General, who is both a barrister and a member of the government. The Attorney General at the time was a rather curious man called Sir Reginald Manningham-Buller.[59] Manningham-Buller had received a third-class honours degree in law at Oxford, and was intensely disliked in legal circles where he went under the nickname 'Bullying Manner'. Lord Devlin, the trial judge,[60] said of him, 'He could be downright rude but he did not shout or bluster. Yet his disagreeableness was so pervasive, his persistence so interminable, the obstructions he manned so far flung, his objectives apparently so insignificant, that sooner or later you would be tempted to ask yourself whether the game was worth the candle: if you asked yourself that, you were finished'.

From the political point of view, the case presented some difficulties to the government. The NHS was less than ten years old at this time and its creation not yet universally supported by the medical profession. The last thing the government wanted was for a doctor to be hanged. To make matters more confusing, the 10th Duke of Cavendish, who had died suddenly in 1950 in the presence of Bodkin Adams, and just 13 days after the death of Edith Morrell, had been the brother-in-law of the Prime Minister, Harold Macmillan.

Against normal practice, prior to Bodkin Adams' arrest,

---

59 His daughter, Eliza Manningham-Buller, subsequently became the first Director General of MI5. Sir Reginald Manningham-Buller later became Lord Chancellor, and became Viscount Dilhorne.

60 Lord Devlin subsequently wrote a book about the case, 'Easing the Passing'; it was the first time that a trial judge had written a book about a case over which he had presided.

Manningham-Buller arranged a secret meeting with the British Medical Association (BMA), at which he is said to have shown them a summary of the police evidence. It has been suggested that this dossier was immediately leaked to the defence legal team. To the surprise of the police, Manningham-Buller decided that it was to be the case of Edith Morrell which was prosecuted, the case in which they considered the evidence to be weakest. Later, the name of Bobbie Hullett was added to the charge sheet.

So, on 18th December 1956, Bodkin Adams was charged that he 'feloniously, wilfully and with malice aforethought did kill and murder Edith Alice Morrell', to which he was said to have replied, 'Murder? Can you prove it was murder? She was dying in any event.'

Bodkin Adams appeared at Eastbourne Magistrates' Court in January 1957, and was remanded in custody pending his trial at the Old Bailey, which began on 18th March. Remarkably, while he was in prison awaiting trial, he received a further £500 in the will of yet another grateful patient.

At the Old Bailey trial, Manningham-Buller was supported by another senior barrister, Melford Stevenson QC, who later became a High Court judge. Melford Stevenson's views on law and order may be deduced from the fact that his house was called 'Truncheons'. He had a robust, no-nonsense, style. He was the judge in the 1969 murder trial of the notorious gangsters, Ronnie and Reggie Kray, who were convicted of killing two petty criminals, George Cornell and Jack 'the Hat' McVitie. Afterwards, he remarked that the only time in the trial Reggie Kray had told the truth was when he had called one of the barristers 'a fat bastard'.

However, in 1955, just two years before the Bodkin Adams case, Melford Stevenson had acted for the defence in the murder trial of Ruth Ellis, a nightclub hostess, who was convicted of killing her boyfriend, a racing driver called David Blakely, with whom she was in a violent and abusive relationship. Ellis was found guilty and, as was law at the time, sentenced to hang, becoming the last woman to be hanged in Britain. It was a deeply shocking case, which certainly did much to hasten the abolition of the death sentence. The trial judge, Sir Cecil Havers,[61] wrote to the Home Secretary recommending clemency, and received a curt rejection. Melford Stevenson had been, perhaps uncharacteristically, deeply moved by the case, believing that the grounds for reprieve had been overwhelming. Perhaps he didn't have the stomach for another high profile murder trial.

Bodkin Adams' defence was placed in the hands of Geoffrey Lawrence QC,[62] a distinguished and highly regarded barrister, but who usually acted in real estate and divorce cases, and who had never previously appeared in a murder trial.

In the earlier committal hearings at Eastbourne Magistrates' Court, the magistrates and the prosecution made a serious procedural error, which ultimately was to derail their case. The chairman of the local magistrates, Lt-Col Roland Gwynne, stood down from his role, as he was a patient, personal friend

---

61 Grandfather of the actor, Nigel Havers.

62 Subsequently Sir Geoffrey Lawrence; he should not be confused with another Sir Geoffrey Lawrence who presided over the Nuremburg War Crimes Tribunal in 1946.

and shooting companion of the accused.[63] The bench thus consisted of David Honeysett, a rather jolly local publican; Mary Bradford, the wife of a coal merchant; Eileen Comer, the daughter of a local hotelier; Lionel Turner, the proprietor of the local newspaper and Colonel Leonard Stevens, owner of a local preparatory school. Their role was to establish whether there was a case to be answered, and they were entitled to hear evidence in public or in private but, anxious not to lose their moment in the limelight, opted for a public hearing. It was the intention of the prosecution to bring evidence that the death of Mrs Morrell was part of a pattern of similar deaths, although at this stage Bodkin Adams had only been charged with one murder.

Geoffrey Lawrence, ever the gentleman, asked the magistrates to retire so that he could address them privately. He then explained that if evidence was disclosed at this stage of other cases, they might subsequently be ruled inadmissible at trial. The magistrates were slightly out of their depth with these complex legal niceties and left matters to Melford Stevenson, acting for the prosecution, who opted to go back into open court, and promptly blundered into the elephant trap of disclosure, thereby undermining an important element of his case.[64]

At the trial at the Old Bailey, the prosecution case was to rest on the evidence of Edith Morrell's nurses and their

---

63 There were persistent, but entirely baseless, rumours that Gwynne and Bodkin Adams were in a homosexual relationship, and this at a time when homosexual acts were against the law.

64 The Criminal Justice Act 1967 restricted the reporting of committal proceedings in criminal cases; it was prompted by the Bodkin Adams case.

observations of the accused's behaviour, and on their expert witness, Dr Arthur Douthwaite, a senior physician at Guy's Hospital, London. They had also assumed that when it was Bodkin Adams' turn to appear in the witness box, his garrulous nature would lead him to stick his neck in the hangman's noose.

The trial lasted 17 days, at the time the longest murder trial in British legal history.[65] Unable, thanks to the issues in the earlier committal hearings to advance the idea of multiple murders with a similar pattern, the prosecution case was already a weak one. It fell apart further when a member of the defence team was on the same train from Eastbourne as the four nurses who were to give evidence, and overheard them rehearsing what they were going to say in court. When the police had searched Bodkin Adams' home prior to arresting him, they had discovered Mrs Morrell's nursing care records. These had been passed to the prosecution but never read, and then somehow reached the defence team. It was clear that there were major discrepancies between what had been recorded at the time and what the nurses had remembered seven years later, something which the defence was to exploit.

But the real nail in the coffin was the evidence of the expert witness, Dr Douthwaite. He suggested that any doctor who administered a drug to a patient which resulted in their death should be regarded as having murdered them, even if the patient was severely distressed by their symptoms, and likely to die in any case. If this was really true it would be impossible for any doctor to treat a terminally ill patient. Finally, Geoffrey Lawrence decided not to put his client in the witness box,

---

65   The record was subsequently overtaken by the Kray trial.

thereby denying the prosecution the chance to question him.[66] In his closing speech he said: 'Trying to ease the last hours of the dying is a doctor's duty and it had been twisted and turned into an accusation for murder'.

The jury retired for 44 minutes and returned to give a 'not guilty' verdict. Not being able to face the prospect of losing again if the Bobbie Hullett case came to trial, Manningham-Buller showed typical bad grace. The normal procedure would be for the prosecution to announce at the outset that they were offering no evidence, and for the judge to direct the jury to formally bring in a 'not guilty' verdict. Instead, he announced *nolle prosequi*, a device where the Crown suspends prosecution of a case. This can be used legitimately to protect a guilty person granted immunity to turn Queen's Evidence, or in cases where the accused is too ill to stand trial, but had never been used to prevent an acquittal. It did not enhance Manningham-Buller's reputation.

Bodkin Adams was released from prison, where he had been on remand for 14 weeks. The *Daily Express* newspaper, which alone of all the press had taken Bodkin Adams' side during the trial, paid him £10,000 for his story. When Bodkins Adams died in 1983, he left £1000 to the journalist, Percy Hoskins, who had been the paper's crime reporter at the time. Shortly after the story appeared, before his death, the Eastbourne Medical Society wrote to Bodkin Adams demanding his resignation, saying that selling his story to the papers had brought the

---

66   This isn't often done in murder trials, but was a technique also used with success by George Carman QC in his defence of Jeremy Thorpe, the former leader of the Liberal Party on a charge of attempted murder.

medical profession into disrepute. They made no comment on any other aspect of his behaviour.

The police were not yet finished with him, and in July 1957 he appeared at Lewes Assizes charged with a number of offences relating to failing to keep a proper record of his dangerous drugs and for not storing them in a safe manner. It seems likely that his carelessness in this matter was not worse than many other GPs of that era and, indeed, when Harold Shipman first went to Todmorden in 1974 he seemed to have inherited a similar recklessness of record keeping and storage of dangerous drugs.[67] There was a further additional charge of selling NHS elasticated stockings to a private patient, hardly the most heinous of crimes.

By this time, Bodkin Adams was exhausted by the whole business, and so he accepted the advice of his legal team to plead guilty and subsequently received a hefty fine. All criminal convictions of doctors are reported to the GMC who determines whether a disciplinary hearing is required. Whereas in the case of Harold Shipman, who in 1976 had been convicted of multiple drug offences (see Chapter 4), they had deemed that no action was necessary, Bodkin Adams was called to a disciplinary hearing on 27th November 1957 and his name was erased from the Medical Register. In fact, he was reinstated three years later and after a further year was permitted to once again prescribe and administer dangerous drugs.

What does seem remarkable is that the GMC gave no thought as to how widespread the deficiencies of care were

---

67   See Chapter 4 'Where There's a Will There's a Way'.

that Bodkin Adams had demonstrated. His record keeping was poor, but was it any worse than that of many GPs in that era? The prescribing of barbiturates to Bobbie Hullett was reckless and inappropriate, but in the 50s the misuse of these drugs was widespread and worsened in the 60s.[68] Bodkin Adams had an eccentric style of practice, albeit one that was much loved by his patients, but at the time there were so many GPs who worked single-handed that it was easy for mavericks to behave as they wished, as Harold Shipman was to demonstrate some 30 years later. Perhaps most importantly, the way in which opiate drugs were used by GPs with minimal record keeping was probably widespread, and was still being exploited by Harold Shipman.

If the GMC had, as it should have, taken a wider view of the safety issues that had been revealed by Bodkin Adams, it is highly likely that the Shipman case would have been averted, as might the explosive spread of medically generated barbiturate addiction.

Harold Shipman remains the only doctor to have been convicted of murdering a patient. However, given the prominent role of wills in the cases of Shipman, Alemi and Bodkin Adams, perhaps in place of the elaborate and ineffective process of appraisal and revalidation that the GMC have introduced, they should merely ask doctors each year whether they have been in receipt of a legacy from a grateful patient.[69]

However, most importantly, after the Bodkin Adams case, the GMC should have attempted to define how doctors can or

---

68 In 1962, the film star, Marilyn Monroe, died of a barbiturate overdose.

69 In 45 years as a doctor I have never been the beneficiary of a patient's will.

cannot legitimately ease the symptoms of gravely ill patients but, again, neither they, nor anyone else, had the courage to offer guidance. It was certainly the view of Lord Devlin, the trial judge, that Bodkin Adams had killed patients, but the open question was as to whether or not he had murdered them. No-one seemed willing to step into this moral, political and legal minefield, and the result was that there have been two further murder trials of doctors in relation to treatment given to distressed and dying patients when there was no prospect of recovery, Dr Leonard Arthur, a consultant paediatrician, in 1981, and Dr David Moor, a GP, in 1999. Both were acquitted.

> *In his closing speech to the jury in Dr Arthur's case (he had ordered 'nursing care only' together with a mild sedative in a newborn child with multiple severe congenital abnormalities, including of the brain), his barrister, George Carman QC, said: 'He could, like Pontius Pilate, have washed his hands of the matter. He did not, because good doctors do not turn away. Are we to condemn him as a criminal because he helped two people [the mother and child] at the time of their greatest need? Are we to condemn a doctor because he cared?'* [70]

Leonard Arthur died of a brain tumour in 1983 at the age of 57, just two years after his acquittal.

After Dr Moor had been found not guilty (he had given diamorphine to an elderly man with disseminated cancer who was in great distress), the broadcaster, Ludovic Kennedy, a

---

70 George Carman QC died in January 2001. His obituary in *The Guardian* of 3rd January 2001 is well worth reading.

well-known campaigner for euthanasia, said: 'Dr Moor should never have been tried, the whole trial was a complete waste of time and money. He was only doing what hundreds and hundreds of doctors do in this country every year.'

Neither case would have come to trial if the GMC had provided proper guidance after the Bodkin Adams case. Doctors providing end of life care remain in jeopardy because of the capricious way in which the law can be applied.

Bodkin Adams died in 1983 having broken his hip whilst out shooting. His funeral service, at Holy Trinity Church, Eastbourne, was attended by some 180 friends and former patients, and the vicar, the Revd Kenneth Blyth, spoke of his devout faith, his sincerity and his charitable work. As a final postscript, in 1991 the Eastbourne District General Hospital was looking for a name for its new private practice unit. A local GP, Dr Tim Gietzen, proposed that it should be called *The John Bodkin Adams Wing*. He wrote, 'Not only is he Eastbourne's most famous doctor, but the name will encapsulate the spirit in which the NHS is now being managed'. His helpful suggestion was not adopted.[71]

---

71 In 1986, BBC TV showed a docudrama of the story, *The Good Doctor Bodkin Adams*, written by Richard Gordon (himself a doctor) who had been the author of the 'Doctor in the House' books. Timothy West was remarkably convincing in the role of Bodkin Adams.

CHAPTER 6

Shoot the Messenger

From when he was a young boy growing up in Kenya, Alban Barros D'Sa[72] always dreamed of becoming a doctor. Family circumstances meant that he had to leave school at 16 and work to support his parents and help his younger siblings complete their education. When he was 23, he came to London, and worked while he studied for his A levels at evening classes in West Ham. He obtained a place to study medicine at Bristol and worked night shifts in a factory to pay his way. He was an outstanding student, winning prizes in surgery, obstetrics, ENT and ophthalmology. On graduation in 1967, he was awarded the Brocklehurst Prize, given to the outstanding student of the year.

He trained in surgery and was appointed consultant surgeon at Walsgrave Hospital (now University Hospital Coventry – see later), in 1979. Initially, he specialised in general and vascular surgery, but in the mid-80s there was the exciting new development of laparoscopic ('keyhole') surgery. This was a major advance in that operations on the gallbladder and bowel could be performed through much smaller skin

---

72   His name derives from his ancestry in Goa, formerly a Portuguese colony in Western India.

incisions, resulting in far shorter hospital stays for patients. He travelled to the United States for training in the technique and became the first surgeon at the hospital to adopt it. For someone who had experienced such a tortuous journey to becoming a doctor, it was not surprising that he was utterly dedicated to his patients and to his work, and was an enthusiastic teacher of medical students and junior doctors.[73]

From the 1950s onwards, it had become common practice in hospitals, especially in surgical departments, for regular meetings to be held for cases to be discussed in which there had been an unexpected or unfavourable outcome. The format varied from place to place and they were sometimes given the rather gruesome name of 'death and disaster' meetings, but they were intended as a blame-free learning opportunity. From the late 1980s these became more formalised into what was called 'clinical audit', in which it was intended that results should be measured against national standards. Such analysis needs to be done carefully. It is perfectly possible, for example, that one surgeon might have a higher operative mortality than his colleagues if he was operating on more complex cases, on patients who had other serious illnesses or who were older and, therefore, frailer. Conversely, unless care is taken, it would be all too easy for a surgeon to present himself as having superior results to his colleagues by choosing only to operate on younger, fitter patients with less serious problems.

The widespread use of clinical audit coincided with the

---

73   His obituary in *The BMJ* described him as 'a caring, astute, precise, meticulous surgeon; a dedicated individual with a strong will and uncompromising high standards'.

general adoption of keyhole surgery. The surgical skills required in it are very different from those of conventional 'open' abdominal surgery, and whilst the great majority of surgeons adapted quickly, some did not. In some cases, this could be remedied by further training, or by limiting their surgical repertoire to cases where keyhole surgery was not indicated, but inevitably there were a small number of instances where senior surgeons lacked the insight to recognise that they did not have the requisite skills in this new surgical landscape.

In 1999, Alban D'Sa and two of his surgical colleagues realised that one of the four surgeons at Walsgrave who undertook colorectal (lower bowel) surgery had a rate of complications and deaths for elective (i.e., non-emergency) surgery four times the national average. To make life more difficult, the surgeon in question was the Clinical Director for this surgical service, having been appointed to the role by the long-standing Chief Executive, David Loughton. The usual first step in this situation would be for the surgeon's colleagues to discuss the problem with the surgeon in question. Had he just been unlucky in having a run of unusually difficult cases? Did he feel that he needed some more training in laparoscopic techniques? Was there evidence of health or personal issues impacting on his performance? But if nothing could be found to explain matters, or if the surgeon was unwilling to engage, the next step would be to advise the hospital's Medical Director and Chief Executive.

Alban D'Sa and another of his consultant colleagues, Miss Briony Ackroyd, brought their concerns to the attention of David Loughton, the Chief Executive. From the perspective of the Walsgrave's Chief Executive, this was an important time.

The University of Warwick was to open a new medical school in 2000, and as part of this, a new hospital was to be built in Coventry to replace the Walsgrave and to be the clinical hub of the medical school. The last thing he wanted was anything that reflected badly on their clinical services.

They might reasonably have expected Mr Loughton to arrange an external review, perhaps organized through the Royal College of Surgeons, and possibly with the duties of the consultant in question being restricted until such a review had been completed. What they did not anticipate, however, was that the Chief Executive took no action against the apparently underperforming surgeon, who was allowed to continue operating with no restrictions on his practice, and suspended Mr D'Sa and Miss Ackroyd from duty (on full pay), to face a disciplinary enquiry. Miss Ackroyd was further reported by Mr Loughton to the GMC in respect of 30 cases of alleged professional incompetence. All were investigated by the GMC and rejected as being without substance. At the conclusion of the GMC's inquiry, they recommended that she should be allowed back to work, which Mr Loughton refused to agree to. She finally left the hospital in 2003 with a substantial financial settlement.

In the meantime, after seven months in which he had been unable to work, Mr D'Sa attended a disciplinary meeting at the hospital. He was given a warning as to his behaviour, but was still not allowed to return to work, as Mr Loughton further accused him of a breach of confidentiality in having written to his MP, Jim Cunningham (as he was fully entitled to have done), in 1999, drawing his attention to the patient safety issues at Walsgrave relating to the excessive death rates in surgery relating to one of the surgeons. Meanwhile, quite remarkably, David Loughton had, in 2000, been awarded a CBE for services to healthcare.

The British Medical Association (BMA), acting for Alban D'Sa, took the hospital to the High Court, and won a judgement that he should be allowed back to work. David Loughton still refused to accept this and brought an appeal, which was rejected. The hospital's legal costs are thought to have been around £500,000. On 27th March 2001, Geoffrey Robinson,[74] another of Coventry's MPs, raised the situation in the House of Commons, saying: 'It is important to stress that Mr D'Sa's professional competence has not been questioned. No-one claims that he is anything other than a good surgeon. When we are so desperately short of cancer surgeons and others, colorectal work is associated with cancer problems, how can a surgeon of acknowledged competence and with an undisputed professional reputation be left idle for 18 months?'

In May 2001, the consultants at the hospital passed a vote of no confidence in the management and, in June 2001, there was a public meeting in Coventry, organized by Geoffrey Robinson, demanding Mr D'Sa's reinstatement. A petition on his behalf generated over 8,000 signatures.

In July 2001, Alban D'Sa finally returned to work. Dozens of his consultant colleagues lined up outside the hospital to applaud him on his first day back. He explained at the time that

---

74 Geoffrey Robinson was an MP for 43 years, and briefly Minister under Tony Blair. He had had a highly successful career as a businessman prior to entering Parliament, which gave him considerable credibility within the Labour Party.

his only concern was that he should be allowed back before his scheduled retirement date in spring 2002. But meanwhile, the people of Coventry had been deprived of his skills for some 20 months whilst he had sat at home on full pay.

But things were not over at Walsgrave. In September 2001, the Commission for Health Improvement (CHI), a new NHS healthcare inspectorate that had only been established in 1999, issued a damning report giving the hospital a 'zero-star rating' (the lowest available). Among its many criticisms was that there had been a breakdown in communication between the management and the consultant staff. Meanwhile, evidence was emerging of an excessive mortality rate in cardiac surgery cases at the hospital.

On the day that the CHI report was released, the six MPs whose constituencies were served by Walsgrave called for the Chief Executive's resignation. In November 2001, they secured a debate in Parliament on the situation at the hospital, and again demanded his resignation, firmly placing responsibility for the hospital's plight on his shoulders. On the morning of the debate, the Chairman of the hospital, Gary Reay, a former purchasing director at the car company, Peugeot, resigned live during an interview on the BBC local radio station, but not before heaping praise on David Loughton.

In the debate in the House of Commons, Geoffrey Robinson pulled no punches. I reproduce his speech in full (from Hansard), because it lays bare the extraordinary situation that the hospital found itself in:

'I congratulate my hon. Friend the Member for North Warwickshire (Mr. O'Brien) on securing this debate. It is an important debate for those who live in Coventry and in the other constituencies whose MPs strongly associate themselves with what has been said today, because the health of the area is at stake.

'As my hon. Friend said, the debate is directly and inescapably about the chief executive, Mr David Loughton. None of us takes it lightly on ourselves to criticise—let alone call for the resignation of—a chief executive by name, bearing in mind the privileges that we have. Those privileges must be respected all the more because they are unique in what they enable us to do and say in the House. For that reason, I would like to say that in no way does the siting of the new PFI hospital—much though we disagreed on it—have anything to do with the lack of confidence that we now have in the chief executive. It was already evident when we were debating that matter, when we disagreed with Mr Loughton, that it was impossible to reason with the man, and that he was arrogant and dismissive.

'That was a couple of years ago and, far from getting better, things have got worse. We saw that in the case where Mr Loughton attempted to abuse correspondence between my hon. Friend the Member for Coventry, South (Mr Cunningham) and one of his constituents, a distinguished consultant surgeon at the hospital. Mr Loughton tried to use a letter as a reason for suspending, confirming the suspension of, and obtaining the dismissal of that fine, distinguished surgeon. Mr Loughton would not listen to reason. He went to the high court, then to a higher court still. Each time his *arguments were demolished, and each time he had to run away in shame, all at a cost to the long-suffering taxpayers of Coventry of £250,000.*

'*Straight after that came the CHI report, casting disgrace on the management of the hospital. The very thought that one could leave the person who had been in charge for 10 years and brought the hospital to that state of affairs in charge for another three months to turn it round defies any logical analysis. After that, we had the report on coronary bypass surgery. There may be arguments on both sides there, but it is interesting that the hospital should have come bottom of the league in that field—a field that the chief executive had boasted was the jewel in the crown of Walsgrave hospital.*

'*In the light of Mr Loughton's behaviour in referring in open meetings at the hospital to some of his staff as the five on his hit list whom he is determined to get rid of, naming them, and referring to them using dismissive and abusive language, it is scarcely surprising that the very people that he needs—that any manager would need—to turn round the hospital after ten years of his mismanagement have passed a vote of no confidence in him. Sixty-six per cent have said that they have no confidence in him. How could anyone turn round a hospital with sixty-six per cent of the staff against him? The hospital has no personnel director, and it cannot recruit a medical director—no one will take on the job—or new consultant surgeons. There is not a grade A consultant in the building, and it would need one to become a teaching hospital.*

'*The whole of the management is dysfunctional.*

Therefore, any details of a change in the chairmanship of the hospital that the Minister might give us today will be an irrelevance, and cannot be used as a sop to deflect us from the primary objective of obtaining a new chief executive.

'If we do not succeed with the Minister today, we shall take the matter to our right hon. Friend the Secretary of State and to the chief executive of the NHS. We shall not let up. If we have to, we shall—in the best of traditions—call another public meeting in Coventry, at which it will be absolutely clear where the chief executive stands, not in terms of our estimation or our sense of confidence, but in the estimation of the people he is meant to serve. I hope that it will not come to that. I hope that the Minister, the Department and the executive of the NHS will see that this situation can be resolved only by taking the simple step of replacing the chief executive.'

In December 2001, the management at Walsgrave Hospital finally received a report from the Royal College of Surgeons into colorectal surgery, recommending that the surgeon who had been the subject of Miss Ackroyd and Mr D'Sa's original complaint, Mr Habib Kashi, should no longer undertake rectal surgery. The report was leaked to the *Birmingham Post* newspaper, and shortly afterwards the new Chairman of the hospital board, Bryan Stoten, announced that 'if the culprit was found he would be sacked'. One would form the impression that he was more concerned by the image of the hospital than the potential harm to patients. It had only taken two-and-a-half years for the necessary action to be taken.

On 5th March 2002, David Loughton finally resigned as

Chief Executive, but not before he had suspended another consultant, Dr Raj Mattu, whose case would reverberate for several years, and ultimately cost the NHS more than £10 million, as well as depriving the hospital of the services of an outstanding consultant for some eight years.

Later that month, the situation at Walsgrave was the subject of another debate in Parliament. The verbatim account can be read in the on-line version of Hansard.[75] It is a depressing account of the damage done by a relentlessly bullying management. In the course of the debate, James Plaskett, MP for the neighbouring constituency of Warwick and Leamington, commented: 'Will the Minister comment on what she thinks should happen to chief executives who have such a record on leaving their post? Should they pop up in due course, elsewhere in the National Health Service?'

In a similar vein, Geoffrey Robinson, one of his fellow Coventry MPs, addressed the same subject: *'In passing, I address the question of Mr Loughton's resignation. I ask respectfully what the redundancy arrangements will be. Will there be severance pay or will he move to another position in the NHS? The Minister may not be able to give an answer this morning, but the people of Coventry have a considerable interest in knowing what is going to happen.'*

Earlier, he had expressed the opinion that Mr Loughton should have been dismissed rather than having been allowed to resign.

---

75 www.hansard.parliament.uk/commons/2002-03-20/debates.

Another local MP, Andy King, the member for Rugby and Kenilworth (an area served by Walsgrave Hospital), also expressed the view that the Chief Executive should have been sacked, and that this should have been done much sooner.

The local MPs must have had some sixth sense about the situation, because two years later David Loughton was appointed as the new Chief Executive at the Royal Wolverhampton Hospital (RWH), just 34 miles down the road from his old job. The RWH was a hospital which had run into severe financial problems and was being forced to cut services in an attempt to balance its books. His arrival was greeted by the hospital's Chairman like that of a latter-day Messiah. Professor Mel Chevannes, chairman of the Royal Wolverhampton Hospitals NHS Trust, said, 'David Loughton brings with him a great wealth of experience at top level management, both within the NHS and the private sector'. But leopards don't change their spots and, predictably, acrimony, suspensions, pay outs and employment tribunals followed in due course.

If the treatment of Miss Ackroyd and Mr D'Sa had been inexcusable, the story of their colleague at Walsgrave, Dr Raj Mattu, proved to be a masterclass in the abuse of power by NHS managers.

Dr Mattu qualified in medicine from the University of Cambridge and trained to be a cardiologist. Throughout his training he showed himself to be an assiduous and highly talented doctor, and he did important research on genetic factors in heart disease. He could well have been appointed to a professorial post at one of the top London teaching hospitals, but in 1998 he was headhunted by Walsgrave Hospital, and the opportunity to take up a consultant appointment in his native Coventry was something that he could not resist. An additional attraction was his involvement in the new medical school at the University of Warwick, which would have its clinical students train at the hospital,[76] and he was offered the possibility of research laboratories on the university campus, for which he had been awarded a large research grant.

Soon after he started working at Walsgrave, Dr Mattu became concerned about dangerous working practices in the cardiology department. One particular concern was the hospital management's insistence in trying to increase capacity by having five beds in cardiology bays which had been designed for four patients. This resulted in occasions when it was impossible to reach patients who required emergency cardiac resuscitation. After an episode when he had been present when a 35-year-old man had died on the ward when the configuration of the beds prevented access for the cardiac arrest trolley, Dr Mattu and two senior nurses made a serious incident report. Dr Mattu had a series of meetings with senior managers, but to no avail. In 2001, the consultants in the cardiology department passed a vote of no confidence in the clinical director and the directorate manager, and chose Dr Mattu to be their new director.

The 2001 report by CHI criticised the five-bed policy and demanded that it ended at once. It highlighted the high death

---

76 Despite its name, the University of Warwick is located on the outskirts of Coventry.

rate for patients at the hospital[77] and noted a 'climate of fear' among clinicians created by senior management, which deterred clinicians from raising safety issues. David Loughton rejected their concerns. To make matters worse, although conversations between clinicians and CHI inspectors were intended to be strictly confidential, under pressure from David Loughton, they revealed to him Dr Mattu's name as one of their sources, although it was only much later that Dr Mattu learned this.

Finally, after detailed discussions with the BMA and the GMC, and with their approval, Dr Mattu gave an interview with BBC Radio 4 at which he brought his concerns over patient safety at Walsgrave to public attention. At every stage, he had acted correctly and had only gone public when every other avenue had been exhausted.

Clearly, Mr Loughton perceived Dr Mattu as a threat. The subsequent employment tribunal, held in Birmingham in 2014, found that Mr Loughton had used the words to colleagues at the hospital, 'Don't worry, as far as Raj (Dr Mattu) is concerned, we are not worried about a parking ticket, we want to get him off the road completely'. Shortly afterwards, Dr Mattu was suspended on full pay pending a disciplinary hearing. Whilst under oath before the 2014 tribunal, Mr Loughton had to admit he had lied and had known all along that the patient deaths had related to overcrowding that Dr Mattu had raised.

In 2005, over three years after Dr Mattu's suspension, the

---

77 An analysis by Professor Sir Brian Jarman of Imperial College London indicated that the 'excess death' rate at Walsgrave actually exceeded that at Stafford Hospital, which has always been regarded as marking the low watermark of NHS practice.

hospital finally conducted a disciplinary hearing under an external barrister, Andrew Stafford QC, who concluded that there were no grounds for his continuing suspension. The hospital refused to accept this judgement, and his suspension continued.

Eventually, in 2007, after concerted pressure from Dr Mattu's legal team, the suspension was lifted, only to be followed by almost a year of arguments about a programme of 're-skilling' as he had not done any clinical work for several years. The hospital also sent some 200 complaints about Dr Mattu to the GMC querying his fitness to practice. The complaints ranged from the frivolous to the absurd. All were thoroughly investigated by the GMC and found to be baseless. Finally, in 2010, the hospital dismissed Dr Mattu after a further disciplinary hearing, which he had been unable to attend as he was unwell, recovering from a major lung operation.

It took a further four years until Dr Mattu's case came before an employment tribunal, which ruled that Dr Mattu had been unfairly dismissed, and that he had done nothing to cause or contribute to his dismissal. In 2016, he was finally awarded £2.5 million in damages. It has been estimated that the hospital's legal costs amounted to well over £14 million, and that, in addition, they had spent substantial sums on the services of a PR agency and a private detective in the vain attempt to find evidence to discredit Dr Mattu. Perhaps the greatest cost is that the NHS and the people of Coventry had been denied the services of a highly talented doctor, whose only crime was that he had wished to improve patient care and avoid unnecessary loss of life. Just as concerning is the comment made in 2018 in an article that he wrote for the *Daily Telegraph*: 'Given there is still a lack of independent protection for staff who speak the truth, I cannot presently advise anyone with concerns to come forward.'

Meanwhile, at the Royal Wolverhampton Hospitals, David Loughton was continuing to demonstrate his usual management style.

Sandra Haynes-Kirkbright, known to her friends as 'Sandie', was originally from Texas, and had graduated from the University of Louisiana, before she finally moved to the West Midlands. In 2011, she was appointed 'head of clinical coding and data management' at the Royal Wolverhampton Hospitals NHS Trust, on a salary of £54,000 per annum. She had previously worked in the coding department at Stafford Hospital a place not without its own problems for four years, on about half the salary.

Clinical coding is one of those boring but vital activities which performs an essential function in hospitals of which most people are blissfully unaware. NHS hospitals get paid by the amount of clinical work they do. For example, there will be a 'tariff' for a hip replacement operation, but there will be a higher payment if there is some factor which makes the operation or aftercare more complex, such as if the patient has insulin-dependent diabetes, serious heart disease or if there has been previous hip surgery. Accurate coding is vital for a hospital's income, and in addition coding departments will generate the data upon which evidence of safety, such as re-admission rates and death rates, are computed.

It was not long before Sandie began to notice things that

did not appear to be right. Some of the coding 'appeared to have no other purpose than to increase the income of the Trust'. Furthermore, there seemed to be unusual practices in the way that palliative care cases were being recorded, and this was having an impact on the calculation of 'excess deaths'.[78] The death rate of patients at Wolverhampton, which had previously been worryingly high, suddenly appeared to have fallen. It had always been the case that patients admitted when terminally ill should be excluded from such calculations, because there would be a risk that hospitals would have a disincentive to admit them, but she had discovered that at Wolverhampton all cases who had been notified to the palliative care team were included in this category. This would clearly make the figures look much better, even though many cancer (and other) patients are referred to the palliative care service as a precautionary measure, even if they are not at that stage requiring such care.[79]

The idea that data can be manipulated will come as no surprise to any reader who has worked in the NHS in recent years, but perhaps I can give an example from my own experience and observation. A few years ago, Accident and Emergency Departments (A&E) were mandated that patients must be seen and either discharged or admitted to hospital within four hours. It was a commendable idea, but what would happen to patients who required admission but for whom there was no bed available? One hospital in which I was working, had the bright idea of converting half of the A&E department into an 'acute admissions ward'. The idea was that patients would be

---

78   See Chapter 9 – 'Stafford' where the same thing was going on.

79   Deaths at the Royal Wolverhampton recorded as being 'palliative care' rose from 2% in 2009 to 20% in 2011, while the number of 'excess deaths' (which excluded palliative care cases) fell by 13%.

tended by the same doctors and nurses as in A&E and wait for a space on a 'real' ward, but for the purposes of those counting the numbers, they wouldn't be breaching the four-hour target. This seemed fine, but I did politely point out that on the acute admissions ward, patients were being nursed in 'mixed sex' bays, and this was against the rules, not to mention an affront to patient dignity, especially as it required men and women to be sharing toilet facilities.

The hospital management thanked me for pointing this out, and by the next day they had changed the signage so that this was no longer the 'acute admissions ward' but the 'acute admissions unit'. As it was no longer a ward, the rules on 'mixed sex' wards apparently did not apply. It was one of the rare occasions in my career in the NHS when I was lost for words.

When Sandra Haynes-Kirkbright aired her concerns to managers, their main response seemed to be to ignore them. An external inspection of the hospital was due, and the instructions from David Loughton were to keep Ms Haynes-Kirkbright away from the inspectors and to 'kick this into the long grass'. In frustration, she approached a national newspaper, the *Daily Mail*, which, in March 2013, carried her story under the title 'Hospital hired me to fiddle death figures; expert claims NHS ordered cover-up'.[80]

The hospital responded by suspending her on full pay, a suspension which continued for over four years. In 2013, the Health Secretary, Jeremy Hunt, demanded that the hospital

---

80 https://www.dailymail.co.uk/news/article-2286770/Expert-claims-NHS-ordered-cover-Hospital-hired-fiddle-death-figures.html

discontinue any disciplinary action (the Trust ignored him), and ordered an independent inquiry. This was commissioned by the NHS Trust Development Authority (NHSTDA), and conducted on their behalf by a private company, Verita, at a cost of nearly £200,000. Their report was completed in 2015, but a year of (expensive) legal wrangling followed as to whether its contents could be made public.

The Verita report, when it finally appeared, pulled no punches as to the behaviour of David Loughton and the senior management at the Royal Wolverhampton NHS Trust but, as ever, criticism seemed to be like water off a duck's back. Simon Burns MP, who had been a junior health minister and had previously called for David Loughton's resignation, was reported in the *Daily Mail* as saying: 'It is a disgrace. It is incomprehensible that someone who was removed from their job 12 years ago because of their attitude to whistle-blowers and poor performance should then, like a revolving door, end up working again in the NHS on a high salary.'

But David Loughton was still not without his admirers. Gary Reay (who, you will remember, was Chairman of the Walsgrave NHS Hospitals Trust until 2001), said that Mr Loughton would get rid of anyone who crossed him, comparing him to former Manchester United manager, Sir Alex Ferguson. 'Like Fergie when Jaap Stam, Ruud van Nistelrooy and Roy Keane started getting too big for their boots, David would get rid of anybody he considered a threat, unproductive or disloyal. He had no compulsion moving them out', he said. 'What I liked about him was he was very hard working and had a good sense of humour, and nobody f***** him over. He's an in-your-face tough guy who could, if you let him, bully.'

If a friend said that, one can only imagine what some of his enemies must have said about him.

Not content with suspending Sandra Haynes-Kirkbright on full pay for years on end, David Loughton did the same to a distinguished cancer specialist at Wolverhampton, Professor David Ferry, when he had the temerity to question some doubtful and dangerous practices in patients undergoing chemotherapy at the hospital. Rather than attempt to tackle the issues raised he chose to suspend Professor Ferry and embroil him in a campaign of vilification. As with Dr Mattu before him, the GMC found no evidence to support Mr Loughton's allegations, and eventually, after four years, Professor Ferry decided to move to a prestigious appointment in the United States researching new anti-cancer drugs; yet another able doctor whose services were lost to the NHS.

In April 2019, the University of Wolverhampton awarded David Loughton an honorary doctorate in recognition of his services to healthcare. He remains the longest serving Chief Executive in the NHS. No doubt a generation of aspiring young NHS managers will study his career and seek to model themselves on him. It is an interesting prospect.

CHAPTER 7

In the Soup

Dame Jill Knight was Conservative MP for Edgbaston, Birmingham, from 1966 to 1997. With her blue-rinsed hair, always impeccably coiffured, she had a striking appearance and was not a lady to be trifled with. She had a reputation of being somewhere politically well to the right of Genghis Khan, but she had a particular passion for the rights of patients in the NHS. I met her once when I gave a lecture to a patient support charity of which she was the chairman; she was utterly charming and it was clear her mind was razor sharp. In 1997, when she finally stood down as an MP, she was elevated to the House of Lords with the title of Baroness Knight of Collingtree in the county of Northamptonshire.

One of Lady Knight's particular concerns was of unjust suspensions of doctors in the NHS. A specific case that had exercised her was that of Dr Bridget O'Connell, a consultant paediatrician at King George Hospital in Ilford, Essex. Dr O'Connell had been suspended on full pay in December 1982 and forbidden to set foot on any NHS premises in the district. Her suspension lasted for over 11 years, until May 1994, when all allegations and disciplinary action were withdrawn. Her employers paid her a substantial sum in damages and her legal costs. Even more concerning than the enormous financial cost, of course, was the loss of a caring and competent doctor to the NHS, for over a decade. No disciplinary action was ever taken against any NHS manager who had initiated or sustained the whole absurd process; indeed, their names have never been made public. Dr O'Connell returned to her native Ireland to resume her work as a consultant paediatrician.

What had Dr O'Connell done to warrant such draconian treatment? She had, for several years, tried to raise her concerns with the hospital management about what she regarded as 'dangerous deficiencies in the care of sick children' at the hospital, which she believed were putting young lives at risk. Her anxiety had been such that she would arrange for some children to be admitted to Great Ormond Street Hospital for the weekend when she was off duty. Among her concerns were that diabetic children were 'punished' 'if their blood sugar levels dropped, there was no follow-up of children with suspected non-accidental injuries (only a token service existed for the mentally handicapped),[81] and that some very sick babies were not being sent to special care baby units. The response by the management to her concerns, prior to her suspension, was described by Dr O'Connell as 'five years of harassment and intimidation that you would only expect in a Communist country'. There had, at no stage whatsoever, been any suggestion of deficiency in the standard of Dr O'Connell's clinical work, or any suggestion that she posed any threat to patient care.

In 2000, Lady Knight, as she was by then, introduced into

---

81 'Mentally handicapped' was a term in use at that time. Learning disabled is currently preferred.

the House of Lords a proposal for an Act of Parliament, the 'Suspension of Hospital Doctors Bill'. Lady Knight explained that she had no interest in protecting bad doctors, but that she was concerned about the human costs.[82] Alan Milburn, the Health Minister, who, when in opposition had called for reform, rejected Lady Knight's bill, and it failed to progress. But she was not a lady who was easily deterred, and prompted by her persistent pressure, the Government asked the National Audit Office (NAO)[83] to investigate the cost of staff suspensions in the NHS.

The NAO report[84] appeared in November 2003 and was highly critical of both the financial[85] and the human cost of staff suspensions, especially of medical staff. They found that such suspensions rarely related to questions of patient safety or the clinical competence of the individuals concerned, but rather that cases did not appear to follow any procedural order, that they went on for an entirely inappropriate length of time and hardly ever, in the end, resulted in any disciplinary action. They called for urgent change.

In March 2004, the indefatigable Lady Knight, now aged 81, secured a debate in the House of Lords[86] on the subject of the

---

82 Hospital doctors face rising threat of suspension, *British Medical Journal* 8th July 2000, vol 321:72.

83 The National Audit Office was established in 1984 but its various predecessors go back as far as 1559, in the reign of Queen Elizabeth I, when the office of 'Auditor of the imprests' was created.

84 'The Management of Suspensions of Clinical Staff in NHS Hospital and Ambulance Trusts in England' Report by the Comptroller and auditor general.

85 The NAO identified costs of tens of millions of pounds each year, usually expended for no useful purpose.

86 The full text of the debate is recorded in Hansard, 22nd March 2004.

NAO report, and just a few days beforehand, like manna from heaven, another extraordinary case landed in her lap...

Terence Hope was a highly regarded consultant neurosurgeon at the Queen's Medical Centre (QMC), Nottingham, having been head-hunted from his previous consultant appointment in Aberdeen. One day, entirely out of the blue, he found himself 'in the soup'. A hospital manager came to see him and advised him that he was being suspended with immediate effect, pending a disciplinary investigation; his alleged offence was that he had helped himself to an extra portion of croutons for his bowl of soup in the hospital canteen. He was ordered to leave the hospital premises at once, and not to return. Terence Hope has never spoken about this publicly, but his story was front-page news in the national and international press.[87]

In the debate in the House of Lords, Lady Knight fulminated against the injustice caused by the willingness of NHS managers to abuse their powers. She began:

> *'My Lords, I have lost count of the number of times that I have raised in Parliament the disgraceful way in which Britain deals with suspended hospital doctors, but I have been doing so for some 16 years. Successive governments have failed to listen, but one must never give up trying to right a wrong. Where there is rank injustice and a way to end it, one must just keep on trying.*
>
> *'We treat criminals who have committed the worst*

---

87   Gardening leave for doctor in the soup, *Daily Telegraph* 23rd March 2004.

crimes in the calendar—murder, rape, violent assault, robbery, child abuse; any crime one cares to mention— with more justice, compassion and mercy than we treat suspended hospital doctors. I hold no brief for incompetent doctors or those who break the law but, of all doctors accused and suspended, about 92% are subsequently found to be innocent.

'Suspension comes like a bolt from the blue. The doctor is instantly sent home in disgrace and barred from re-entering his hospital. He is not told what he is alleged to have done. He receives no legal aid; he has no lawyer or friend to help him; there is no appeal. He or she has no idea how long that situation will continue. I know of one case where a woman doctor remained suspended for 11 years.

'Since then, a rule has been made that suspension can continue only for what is termed a 'binding time.' But it does not seem very binding to me. Out of 350 suspensions, hospital trusts have adhered to it only twice. Even being suspended for a year or 18 months—the average is two-and-a-quarter years—can mean the end of a career. Medical advance is too fast for gap years.'

She continued in the same vein, before coming to the saga of Terence Hope and his croutons:

'Only this morning, we heard that a hospital trust, which must have been sent those new rules and has certainly had time to read them, suspended a top brain surgeon who took an extra helping of croutons in his soup. Oh, vile crime! Had he been prepared, perhaps, to be a little less keen on croutons, *he would have continued in his job. I find that incredible. In my Daily Mail this morning I read that he has been sitting at home fully paid since last week, no doubt thinking about croutons. Heaven knows how much suffering that has caused and will cause to his patients. Once a doctor is suspended, his return is neither quick and easy nor inevitable.*

'When I heard of this case this morning, I found it incredible. I found it so impossible to believe that I telephoned the BMA, which checked it. I have to tell noble Lords that every word in the Daily Mail report is true.'

The government minister who was charged with responding, Lord Warner of Brockley,[88] the Parliamentary Under-Secretary of State in the Department of Health, suggested, somewhat improbably, that the Department of Health had no influence or control over hospital managers. He also stated that Mr Hope's heinous crime had been caught on CCTV, a fact which had not been mentioned in any of the extensive press coverage and which, therefore, could only have been made known to him by those same hospital managers over whom he had no influence.

However, two days later, the hospital announced that Terence Hope would be returning to work, but not before a number of patients who had been scheduled to have brain surgery performed by him had had to have their operations rescheduled.

Lady Knight ended her speech with some sadly prophetic words:

---

88   Until 1996 he had been Norman Warner, a civil servant.

'I have a dreadful feeling that I shall have to go on for another 16 years pleading the case for doctors who have been suspended, the suffering they are forced to endure and the amount of money that that costs the NHS. Obviously, what the Government have tried to do, no doubt with every good intention, has been utterly useless. Words fail me.'

Sixteen years later, little has changed, and NHS managers continue to waste money and the lives of talented doctors by abusing the suspension process. Lord Warner's perhaps slightly unguarded suggestion that the Department of Health has no control over the actions of hospital managers is an interesting revelation. In 2010, a popular and well regarded colorectal surgeon at Milton Keynes General Hospital,[89] Mr Talib Al-Mishlab, was suspended by the hospital over allegations that he had an unacceptably high complication rate for certain types of bowel surgery.

The suspension dragged on for nearly five years during which time he was on full pay, even though both the GMC and the National Clinical Assessment Service (NCAS) had judged that he should be allowed back to work. A particular point of note was that the surgical complication rate at the hospital for that type of surgery had been no different before his suspension or after it. The local MP became aware of the story and raised the matter with the Department of Health asking how many hospital consultants were currently suspended in the NHS. Extraordinarily, but perhaps unsurprisingly, the answer that the Department of Health sent back was that they had no idea. After five years, during which the NHS was deprived of his

---

89   Now Milton Keynes University Hospital.

services, Mr Al-Mishlab was appointed as a consultant surgeon at Poole Hospital in Dorset, where his surgical skills are widely appreciated and where he is a highly regarded member of the surgical team.

Unfortunately, I could go on with countless other stories of similar absurd and vindictive actions against dedicated doctors and nurses, but I don't want to depress my readers. I would, however, recommend *Whistle in the Wind,* a book written by Mr Peter Duffy, a consultant surgeon, whose only 'offence' had been to try to ensure patient safety at Furness General Hospital. He was eventually paid substantial damages at an employment tribunal and moved to work on the Isle of Man, safely out of reach of the NHS. The book paints a very personal picture of how NHS managers can attempt to ruin the lives of dedicated doctors and nurses.

Just very occasionally, consultants *do* achieve small moral victories, and they are moments to savour. In 2005, I was asked to become Chairman of the Medical Staff Committee at my hospital. It was not as grand a role as it may sound, but it was my duty to advise the Chief Executive of issues where the consultants might have concerns. I took particularly serious matters relating to patient safety to the CEO, but sometimes my observations were not entirely welcome.

The Chairman of the hospital's board was a retired businessman called Ray Rankmore. He had had a successful and diverse career and was a thoroughly engaging man with whom I generally got on well. His office was close to my outpatient clinic and, one day as I passed, he called me in. He quickly came to the point and said, 'In business, if management think there is someone who isn't 100% behind them, they get rid of them, *just like that*. Then he repeated, '*just like that*' for added emphasis. He continued, 'In the NHS, we can't do things quite like that, so we have to do things somewhat differently'. I was then invited to leave. To this day I am not entirely sure what I had done to upset the hospital management, but clearly he had something in mind.

I have always associated the phrase 'Just like that' with the comedian, Tommy Cooper, whose on-stage conjuring tricks always seemed to end in disaster and whose catch phrase it was. I recounted the story to a few of my colleagues over lunch. Unbeknown to me, one of them decided to use his computer skills to add a red fez, Tommy Cooper's trademark prop, to a picture of Mr Rankmore and send it, along with the story, to the local newspaper that printed it on their front page.

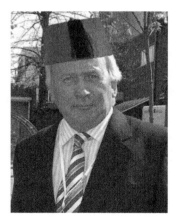

Figure 2. Ray Rankmore.

I claim complete innocence here and, as anyone who knows my total lack of computer skills would attest, I simply would have been incapable of doing it. Mr Rankmore decided that the NHS wasn't for him and resigned shortly afterwards. He had decided that NHS management wasn't his cup of tea. It was a pity because Ray Rankmore was well intentioned and had lots of excellent ideas. In fairness, after this incident, I also decided that any engagement with hospital management wasn't for me and stepped down from my role of Chairman of the Medical Staff Committee.

So, why *do* hospital managers persist in behaving so badly towards doctors? Perhaps the answer lies in the comic novel *Candide, ou l'Optimisme*, written by the French writer, Voltaire, in 1759. In the course of the book, Candide witnesses the execution of a British officer by firing squad, and it is explained to him that 'in this country, it is good to kill an admiral from time to time to encourage the others'.[90]

Voltaire's observation was based on the true case of Admiral Byng who, just two years earlier, had been subject to a court marshal and shot by a firing squad of marines. In the early part of the 'Seven Years' War', Byng, as commander of the Royal Navy (RN) in the Mediterranean, was ordered to assemble a fleet and sail to Minorca to secure it against a possible French assault. Byng wrote to his superiors stating that several of the ships were unprepared and those that were fit to sail were undermanned, but he was ordered to set sail nevertheless. He stopped in Gibraltar, where the garrison commander refused his request for further supplies and a contingent of marines, and set off again towards Minorca. A rather inconclusive battle with

---

90 Dans ce pays-ci, il est bon de tuer de temps en temps un amiral pour encourager les autres.

the French fleet took place off Port Mahon, and Byng decided that his ships should return to Gibraltar for repairs. However, before he could return to battle, instructions were received from the Admiralty that he was to return to England. He was charged with having 'not given his utmost'. Lord Newcastle, the Prime Minister, wrote to a colleague, 'I thought it not fair, to lay the loss expressly upon Byng, though there it will and must be laid, and only there'. Newcastle, and almost everyone else, knew that the *real* problem was the chaotic administration of the Admiralty. The case caused uproar,[91] but Byng was duly executed, the last Admiral to meet this fate. He was buried in the family vault at the All Saints Church, Southill, Bedfordshire, and a plaque reads:

> *To the perpetual Disgrace*
> *of PUBLICK JUSTICE*
> *The Honble. JOHN BYNG Esqr*
> *Admiral of the Blue*
> *Fell a MARTYR to*
> *POLITICAL PERSECUTION*
> *March 14th in the year 1757 when*
> *BRAVERY and LOYALTY*
> *were Insufficient Securities*
> *For the*
> *Life and Honour*
> *of a*
> *NAVAL OFFICER*

---

91 In 2007, 250 years after his execution, Byng's family petitioned the Government for a posthumous pardon; their application was refused. Few governments are ever willing to acknowledge their mistakes. His only public memorial is a pub in Potters Bar named after him.

It would seem that there are still NHS managers who would happily follow the practices of the 18th century Admiralty in blaming others for their own shortcomings, and believe that their behaviour bolsters their position. One wonders if we would be better served if hospital managers adopted a more modern approach to management by addressing their own inadequacies, rather than squandering scarce public money and ruining the lives of able doctors who have much to contribute; but, like Lady Knight, don't hold your breath.

CHAPTER 8

The Heart of the Matter

In 1995, Dr Stephen Bolsin (now Professor), a consultant cardiac anaesthetist at Bristol Royal Infirmary, resigned his position and moved with his family to take up a position as Director of critical care in Geelong Hospital, Australia. His move was a considerable loss to the NHS because Dr Bolsin has become an internationally recognised leader in the field of patient safety, but he felt compelled to move away from the UK. He had a bruising experience in exposing the scandal of paediatric cardiac surgery in Bristol. In truth, not all of his colleagues were sorry to see him go.

After receiving his qualification at University College Hospital (UCH), London, Stephen Bolsin trained in anaesthesia and decided to specialise in cardiac anaesthesia; his training included spells at the Royal Brompton Hospital and the Hospital for Sick Children at Great Ormond Street.

In September 1988, he was appointed to his first consultant post at the Bristol Royal Infirmary, and was immediately struck by the rather dilapidated and outdated facilities for cardiac surgery. The arrangement for paediatric cases was complicated by the fact that their care was split between the Bristol Royal Infirmary, where the cardiac operating theatres were situated, and the Bristol Royal Hospital for Children, where they received the rest of their care (situated next to each other in the city centre). There was no specialist paediatric cardiac surgeon, no paediatric intensive care beds, and too few specialist paediatric intensive care nurses.

More concerning to him, however, was the length of the operations, sometimes taking three times longer than identical operations he had seen undertaken in London. In small babies undergoing cardiac surgery and whom have complex abnormalities of their hearts and great vessels, there is a significant risk of brain damage arising from oxygen starvation during the procedure, and this risk increases with the length of time they are on cardiac bypass.

However, even more concerning were his observations on the number who were dying. These are, of course, seriously ill children and surgery is inevitably a high-risk enterprise, but the number who were dying appeared excessive. He knew that something had to be done, but as 'the new kid on the block' he was not in an easy situation. Perhaps it was his upbringing; his parents had both been Christian missionaries who had met working overseas that had given him the fortitude not to shrink from the challenges he was to face, although it did not always make him popular.

The annual report for the paediatric cardiac surgery department at Bristol for 1989–1990 gave a mortality figure of 37.5% for babies under one that had undergone surgery, compared with the national figure of 18.8%. It was a discrepancy which would be hard to explain by mere chance or bad luck. In August 1990, Dr Bolsin wrote to the Chief Executive of the hospital, Dr John Roylance, to raise his concerns. Dr Roylance was in a rather unusual situation because, although medically qualified and a former consultant radiologist, he had been working in a managerial rather than a medical capacity for the previous ten years. He responded to Dr Bolsin's letter by phoning and advising him that his contribution was both unhelpful and unwanted. Shortly afterwards, Dr Bolsin was called to a meeting by Mr James Wisheart, the senior of the two cardiac surgeons operating on children at Bristol.

James Wisheart was a consultant surgeon of the 'old school' and not a man to be trifled with, a dedicated and hardworking doctor with a somewhat autocratic and unapproachable manner. The son of a Methodist preacher from Enniskillen, he had qualified in medicine from Queen's University Belfast (QUB),[92] in 1962 and had been a consultant cardiac surgeon at Bristol since 1975. He was the Chairman of the hospital consultants' committee, and was just about to become the Medical Director of the hospital in addition to his clinical work; in effect, he was the centre of power within the hospital. Mr Wisheart told Stephen Bolsin in unambiguous terms to keep his opinions to himself and, in particular, not to raise them again with Dr Roylance.

Dr Bolsin and other consultant colleagues in the anaesthetic department began to review outcome data of paediatric cardiac surgery at Bristol and to compare it to national figures, but not all the senior members of the team were supportive. The high mortality in the 1989–1990 annual report could not be explained by some unfortunate statistical quirk, because the

---

92   QUB was also the *alma mater* of Dr Bodkin Adams (see Chapter 5).

figures for the next year showed mortality for children under the age of one undergoing surgery at Bristol of 30%, compared to a national figure of 15.8%.

In December 1991, Ian Hislop, the editor of *Private Eye* magazine, invited a junior hospital doctor (as he then was) and part-time stand-up comedian, Dr Phil Hammond,[93] to start contributing a fortnightly column on medical matters, which has appeared ever since under the title 'Medicine Balls' and the byline 'MD'. By coincidence, Dr Hammond was working in the West Country (though not at that time in Bristol), and had repeatedly heard the cardiac surgery department at Bristol referred to as 'The Killing Fields' or 'The Departure Lounge'. In 1988, Dr Hammond had been a House Physician (the most junior grade of hospital doctor), in Bath. An adult patient was admitted with a dissecting aneurysm of the thoracic aorta and required emergency transfer to a hospital with the facilities for urgent cardiac surgery; Hammond, as most junior, and hence most dispensable member of the team, was delegated to travel with him in the ambulance to give medical assistance *en route*, if required. Before they set off, he asked the consultant why the patient was going to Southampton, a rather circuitous 64 miles away, rather than to Bristol which was only 12 miles in the opposite direction. His innocent question was greeted with a wry smile from his colleagues.

In January 1992, a member of the anaesthetic department

---

93 The full transcript of Dr Hammond's evidence given to the Kennedy inquiry into the Bristol cardiac surgery saga may be read on-line at https://web. archive.org/web/20070928073505/ http://www.bristol-inquiry.org.uk/ evidence/transcripts/day64.htm#99

(not Dr Bolsin)[94] and who knew of Hammond's connection with *Private Eye*, gave him specific and alarming details about the death rate for paediatric patients undergoing cardiac surgery at Bristol; the story was first made public in the 'Medicine Balls' column on 14th February 1992. In essence, there were patients dying at Bristol who may well have survived if they had been operated upon elsewhere. Further articles were to appear in *Private Eye* on 27th March, 8th May, 3rd July, 9th October and 20th November 1992, detailing the situation in Bristol in relation to the paediatric cardiac surgery service. Subsequent articles on the very same subject were to appear over the next 20 years.

In April 1992, Stephen Bolsin met Phil Hammond for the first time, although he apparently was not sure who he was, other than that he was an enthusiastic junior doctor and did not realize that he wrote for *Private Eye*. The following month the 'Medicine Balls' column revealed that the Department of Health had known since 1998 that there was a problem with paediatric cardiac surgery at Bristol. The CMO for Wales, Professor Gareth Crompton, had raised with the Supra Regional Services Advisory Group (SRSAG), a body which directed specialist services such as paediatric cardiac surgery, which are only carried out in a few centres, his concerns about the care of cardiac surgery patients being sent from Wales to Bristol. The subject was also covered in a television programme broadcast by BBC Cymru Wales in June 1987, under the title *'Heart Surgery – The Second Class Service.'*

---

94 Hammond was put under intense pressure when giving evidence to the Kennedy inquiry of 2001 to reveal his source, but stuck to his journalistic principles in not revealing it.

The timing of the article in *Private Eye* was particularly inconvenient for Dr Roylance as the hospital was in the process of applying for an 'NHS Quality Chartermark', another of the bizarre schemes that appear from time to time as a form of work creation for otherwise unemployable NHS managers.[95]

In the summer of 1992, Dr Bolsin was unsuccessful in an application for a post as consultant anaesthetist at Oxford. He remains suspicious that he had been subject to a 'whispering campaign' against his appointment. Meanwhile, the Royal College of Surgeons had been commissioned by SRSAG to prepare a report on specialist paediatric cardiac surgery services. Sure enough, its data demonstrated that the results at Bristol were the worst of the nine centres in the country that undertook this type of surgery. Meanwhile, the Department of Health wrote to Dr Roylance asking for his response to the articles in *Private Eye*. His response, apparently drafted by Mr Wisheart, was that the results in Bristol were comparable to anywhere else. Clearly, Dr Roylance believed in the 'ostrich' style of NHS management, sticking his head firmly into the sand. Likewise, the Department of Health took no steps to verify the facts independently. It appeared more interested in protecting the image of the NHS than finding out exactly what it was doing.

By the following year, Stephen Bolsin had accumulated

---

95   It was one of the brainwaves that appeared in the John Major era, along with the Cones Hotline; this was intended to get drivers to phone in with details of redundant traffic cones, but 17,000 calls in three years resulted in only five sets of cones being removed. It became a byword for pointless government initiatives when it appeared politically expedient to be seen to be 'doing something'. Like the NHS Quality Charter Mark, it was quietly put out of its misery.

enough data to approach Dr Roylance and the senior management of the hospital formally. By this stage, he had the support of his fellow anaesthetists, the Royal College of Surgeons, Dr Peter Doyle, a senior medical officer (SMO) at the Department of Health and Professor Gianni Agnelini, the Professor of Adult Cardiac Surgery at Bristol. As had already been realized, the results from Bristol were the worst in the country and, as a result, children were dying. Dr Roylance still dismissed their concerns. His view was that, in any league, someone had to be at the bottom. It was, by any account, an extraordinary attitude; he was discussing the lives of sick children, not football teams. In fact, there was clear evidence from *every other centre* in the country that their survival figures for children undergoing cardiac surgery was improving year-on-year.

Between 1990 and 1993, James Wisheart carried out 11 hole in the heart operations on babies, and five had died, a mortality rate of 45%. In the case of one specific serious congenital abnormality of the heart, tetralogy of Fallot (TOF),[96] the mortality at Bristol was between 20 and 30%. At Alder Hey Children's Hospital, Liverpool, there had been no deaths in some 130 consecutive cases. Nationally and internationally, there was clear evidence that the best results were achieved in specialist centres undertaking the largest number of cases, and by teams doing purely paediatric cases. The workload at Bristol was not sufficient for the necessary skills to be embedded in the team.

---

96 TOF is a congenital abnormality of the heart characterised by four features (hence 'tetralogy'): obstruction to the pulmonary artery, ventricular septal defect, overriding aorta and hypertrophy of the right ventricle; typically affected children become cyanosed (go blue) on minimal exertion.

The evidence presented by Dr Bolsin should have been overwhelming, but paediatric cardiac surgery carried on. In an 18-month period, Mr Wisheart carried out a further four open-heart operations, all with a fatal outcome; only then did he decide to cease operating.

One surgical operation that Mr Wisheart had been keen to introduce to the Bristol cardiac surgery unit was the 'switch procedure' for transposition of the great vessels (TGV). This is a disorder where the child is born with the pulmonary artery arising from the left ventricle and the aorta arising from the right, but there may be other associated abnormalities. Swapping over the pulmonary artery and the aorta to their correct positions may, to the layperson, sound straightforward, but in a tiny baby, already critical ill and with low levels of oxygen in the blood, it takes very considerable skill and teamwork from the surgeons, anaesthetists, nurses and others. By the early 90s, most centres were achieving a 90% operative survival rate, which was remarkable considering how unwell those babies were and the fact that some of them had additional abnormalities of their hearts and major blood vessels.

At Bristol, this operation was predominantly carried out by Mr Wisheart's colleague, Mr Janardan Dhasmana, the only other consultant cardiac surgeon at the hospital who undertook paediatric surgery. Of 13 babies undergoing the 'switch' operation, nine had died. In fairness to him, Mr Dhasmana was a technically accomplished heart surgeon; his results for adult surgery were entirely acceptable and, after some early deaths, he had arranged to spend time at the cardiac surgery unit at Birmingham for further training in the procedure. In fact, at Mr Wisheart's insistence, the audit figures for heart surgery at Bristol were always published as a whole, rather than separating them out to different surgeons. Mr Dhasmana's figures, judged separately, were as good as most surgeons in the UK, and disguised just how poor Mr Wisheart's were. But Mr Dhasmana had been trained by Mr Wisheart himself and showed unshakeable, if somewhat misguided, loyalty to him.

Under pressure from Professor Agnelini, it was agreed that no more 'switch' operations would be performed until a new specialist paediatric cardiac surgeon was employed. However, in January 1995, an acutely ill 18-month-old baby, Joshua Loveday, was admitted to hospital. He had been born with TGV and was in urgent need of surgery. Mr Wisheart and Mr Dhasmana pressed for the need for an emergency operation, which was listed for 12th January. Dr Bolsin, supported by Professor Agnelini, urged them to transfer the child to another surgical centre, but they were determined to continue.

Dr Bolsin phoned Dr Doyle at the Department of Health the day before the operation who, in turn, late in the evening, phoned Dr Roylance, urging him to ensure that Joshua was *not* operated on at Bristol. Dr Roylance stuck to his usual line that clinical matters were not for the Chief Executive. The fateful operation took place the next day and, sadly, Joshua did not survive. Dr Bolsin resigned his post and began to make arrangements for his move to Australia. Shamefully, Joshua Loveday's parents had never been advised of the poor performance of the paediatric cardiac surgery team or been given the option of his being transferred to a cardiac surgery unit elsewhere, and his father, who had signed the consent form for the procedure, never got over his son's death, and he took his own life two years later. Paediatric cardiac surgery was immediately suspended, a whole *five years* after Dr Bolsin had first raised his concerns.

Two years later in 1997, the GMC charged Mr Wisheart, Mr Dhasmana and Dr Roylance with serious professional misconduct. By this time, Mr Wisheart and Dr Roylance had retired from the NHS, thereby protecting their valuable index-linked pensions. The hearing began in 1998 and lasted seven months, the longest and, at a cost of some £2.2 million, the most expensive in the history of the GMC. All three were found guilty; Mr Wisheart and Dr Roylance being struck off the Medical Register, and Mr Dhasmana being banned from undertaking surgery on children, only being allowed to operate on adults under supervision.[97] In fact, he had not undertaken any surgery on children since Joshua Loveday, and had stated that he had no intention to operate on children in the future.

The judgement was greeted with raucous cries for blood from some quarters of the press and from the Health Secretary, Frank Dobson, who, in an interview on BBC-TV's *Newsnight* programme, had demanded that Mr Dhasmana be struck off the Medical Register. The reaction prompted Professor Agnelini, who had repeatedly raised his concerns numerous times, and five other Bristol consultants, to issue a statement in which they accused governmental and professional regulatory bodies of refusing to take action; they said it was 'disgraceful' that they were now sitting 'in sanctimonious judgment' over the failure of doctors in Bristol.[98] Notwithstanding their pleas,

---

97　Four years later he was allowed to resume adult cardiac surgery; his ability in this aspect of his work had never been questioned.

98　C Dyer. British doctors found guilty of serious professional misconduct. *British Medical Journal* 1998, vol 316:1924.

the managers at Bristol, under pressure from Mr Dobson, sacked Mr Dhasmana.

Dr Roylance took his case to appeal before the Privy Council, arguing that he had been working as a manager, not a doctor, and that what the doctors get up to in a hospital is nothing to do with the Chief Executive. His conviction was upheld. In fact, it was only because he was medically qualified that he had had to appear in public before the GMC. A non-medically qualified Chief Executive in the NHS, and the great majority are not medically qualified, would have been able to quietly slink away, as has happened in many other cases. He must have shown considerable aptitude to have climbed the greasy pole of hospital management and to have achieved his position as Chief Executive in one of the largest hospital trusts in the country, but from everything that has been written about him he seems to have regarded his job description as merely balancing the books. He had, therefore, shown no inclination to involve himself in decisions relating to clinical matters. It was a plainly absurd position, rather like a restaurant manager having no interest in the food being served. He had repeatedly been provided with the most unambiguous evidence over several years that something was gravely wrong and had chosen to do nothing about it.

Mr Wisheart had clearly lacked insight into the deficiencies of paediatric cardiac surgery. To be charitable to him, he *had* been in an ambiguous position, as both the senior consultant paediatric cardiac surgeon and as Medical Director. One of the most important roles of a medical director in a hospital is to address issues of performance. Clearly, once questions had been asked about the outcomes of his *own* surgery, he shouldn't have been allowed to sit in judgement on himself.

Surgeons have something in common with elite sportsmen in that they have taken thousands of hours of training to hone their skills and are often the last to realise when they have passed their peak. This is especially true in Mr Wisheart's area of practice where there had been extraordinarily rapid developments. Anyone who follows sport will have seen stars who just fail to accept that they have passed their best and who have become a slightly embarrassing shadow of their former selves. The lucky ones have friends or managers who encourage them to quit when they are at the top. In medicine, it is all too easy for the penny to drop too late and, if, like James Wisheart, you are seen by your colleagues to be powerful and somewhat aloof, no one is likely to forewarn you.

Some years ago, I was involved, from the safe side of the ropes, with professional boxing. I vividly remember what turned out to be the last fight of a popular champion, Dave 'Boy' Green. His long-time trainer and manager, Andy Smith, who had known Green since he was a child, saw the warning signs that he was past his prime and, at the end of the fifth round, called the referee over and told him that he was withdrawing Green from the fight. He then put his arms round Green and told him that his career as a boxer was over. Dave Green, one of the most fearless boxers any of us had ever known, wept inconsolably, but afterwards, acknowledged that Andy Smith was right. Sadly, James Wisheart did not have an Andy Smith to put an arm round him, the inevitable result of having cultivated a position of absolute power and an aura of unapproachability. If he had, he might have stopped operating sooner.

At the completion of the GMC's deliberations, Dr Richard Smith wrote an editorial in *The BMJ* entitled 'All Changed, Changed Utterly'; the title taken from the line in WB Yeats' poem *Easter, 1916*.[99] 'British medicine will be transformed by the Bristol case', he pronounced. The Secretary of State for Health and Social Care, Frank Dobson, announced that there would be a public inquiry to be chaired by Professor Sir Ian Kennedy, a barrister and academic lawyer specializing in the law and ethics of healthcare. The inquiry cost over £14 million and reported in July 2001; its 540-page work was published as 'The report of the public inquiry into children's heart surgery at the Bristol Royal Infirmary 1984–1995: learning from Bristol'.[100]

Professor Kennedy's report was undertaken in a diligent and meticulous manner. It identified that between 30 and 35 babies died at Bristol who were likely to have survived had they been operated on elsewhere. It was, however, criticised by Laurence Vick, the lawyer who represented many of the parents of children who had been operated on at Bristol, for not having inquired into the cases of brain damage in children who had survived heart surgery at Bristol, which had occurred at a higher rate than in other centres undertaking paediatric cardiology.[101] Mr Vick also drew attention to the impact on

---

99 *British Medical Journal* 1998, vol 316:1917–1918. The full line is 'All changed, utterly changed; a terrible beauty is born.'

100 The on-line version may be accessed at: https://webarchive.nationalarchives.gov.uk/20090811143810/http://www.bristol-inquiry.org.uk/final_report/report/index.htm

101 A number of successful claims relating to post-operative brain damage caused by oxygen deprivation during cardiac surgery were eventually settled; some took 20 years to be resolved, which must have been an additional burden for parents to bear. Laurence Vick has always asserted that the number of affected children was substantially higher than had been acknowledged by the Kennedy report.

families. It wasn't just the father of Joshua Loveday who had committed suicide, four others had.

The report made the obvious conclusion that James Wisheart had 'lacked insight' into his own poor results, had mislead the Trust board and that he had an 'autocratic' style, which did not encourage critical analysis of the cardiac surgery service. Dr Roylance was criticised for having mislead the Department of Health by implying that the Trust board was aware of the problems when they were not, and for failing to seek a review of the service until 1994. With regard to Mr Dhasmana, it concluded that he focused excessively on his own surgical technique rather than looking at the bigger picture. But the report did not confine its criticism to the three individuals who had appeared before the GMC.

Dr Peter Doyle, an SMO at the Department of Health, had been given an envelope by Dr Bolsin containing a detailed audit of the outcome of paediatric cardiac surgery at Bristol and had filed it away unread, an action the report described as 'seriously inappropriate'. Mrs Margaret Maisey had been the Director of Nursing at Bristol, as well as the Director of Operations and Dr Roylance's 'eyes and ears' or, as she described herself, 'the Chief Executive's rottweiler'. Unfortunately, she was not someone whom any of the nursing team would have felt comfortable approaching with concerns.[102]

Norman Halliday, the medical secretary of the SRSAG (the body which allocated Department of Health funding to the specialist units providing paediatric cardiac services), was

---

102 She retired in 1997 with her full NHS pension.

criticised for a complete lack of interest in the outcome of the treatment it was funding, even when specific concerns, such as those of the CMO of Wales, were brought to his attention. Indeed, the lack of interest of the Department of Health and of SRSAG throughout seems remarkable. It was rather as if an on-line shopper doing their weekly food shop just sent a random amount of money and did not trouble to check what turned up on the delivery van.

Sir Terence English, the former President of the Royal College of Surgeons and a cardiac surgeon who had pioneered heart transplantation at Papworth Hospital and who had also been a member of SRSAG, was criticised for not having brought his concerns about Bristol to the attention of the group and its chairman. Dr Hyam Joffe, the consultant paediatric cardiologist at Bristol, who had been head of children's services from 1990 to 1994, was also criticised for not having raised concerns.

The report, whilst attributing blame to the actions (or lack of actions) of some individuals, is clear that it was the system as a whole that had failed, right up to the Department of Health, who 'were not interested in results; they were interested in as many people as possible passing through the system as possible for as low a cost as possible.'

The report presented a bold and optimistic vision for the future, stating 'The culture of the future must be a culture of safety and of quality; a culture of openness and accountability; a culture of public service; a culture in which collaborative teamwork is prized; and a culture of flexibility in which innovation can flourish in response to patients' needs.' It called for steady increases in resources, good leadership, better systems of accountability, explicit standards of care, better management and communication, public involvement at all levels and putting patients first, in deeds not words. But, as Richard Smith, the editor of *The BMJ* pointed out in a response that was broadly supportive, just how this was to be achieved was less clear.[103]

The report made 198 recommendations for the future. Perhaps, with hindsight it would have been better if it had focused on a few key points. Some, such as that the NHS should do more for children, or that members of clinical teams must work together, are self-evidently laudable, but *how*, exactly, was it to be made possible? Others had not been fully thought through; for example, the report asked that data on clinical performance (as in the outcome of paediatric cardiac surgery) should be collected as a matter of routine and made readily available. Surely no one could argue against that, it had been a key failing at Bristol, but what would be the impact in an NHS already working at full capacity? If patients were identified as doing significantly better with hip replacements if these were done in Newcastle than in Penzance, to take a purely hypothetical example, would everyone in the South West want to travel up North for their operation and, if they did, and the service became overwhelmed with numbers, would it still maintain its better results?

One of the most important recommendations, that there should be a single independent national body charged with ensuring safety, was quietly ignored; this was, of course, exactly

---

103 One Bristol, but there could have been many. *British Medical Journal* 2001, vol 323:179–180.

the type of change which had transformed safety in the nuclear industry (see Chapter 2) and the UK railway system, now the safest in the world.

Another recommendation was that there should be some supervision of hospital managers in terms of a system of appraisal and revalidation, as was subsequently introduced for doctors and nurses. It was a suggestion which vanished without trace. A few years later, I approached the head of the school of management at one of our leading universities with the suggestion that they might run a programme for NHS managers leading to a qualification. They were full of enthusiasm, as indeed were managers at my own hospital with whom I had informally discussed the matter, but we never received a reply from the Department of Health.

In the introduction to his report, Professor Kennedy states, 'It would be reassuring to believe that it could not happen again. We cannot give that reassurance. Unless lessons are learned, it certainly could happen again'. Sadly, it did not take long for these prophetic words to be proved correct. In 2004, an academic article appeared in *The BMJ* analysing the outcome of all paediatric cardiac surgery operations in the United Kingdom between 1991 and 2002.[104] The authors included Professor Sir Brian Jarman, who had been a member of the Kennedy report team, and Professor Paul Elliott, who had acted as an expert adviser to the report.

---

104 Paediatric cardiac surgical mortality in England after Bristol: descriptive analysis of hospital episode statistics 1991–2002. *British Medical Journal* 2004, vol 329:825–829.

The paper, which looked at over 11,500 operations, showed that, nationally, there had been a progressive decline in the death rate in children undergoing heart surgery and that, in Bristol, the rate had fallen dramatically after 1995 when a new specialist paediatric cardiac surgeon had been appointed, and by 2002, it was below the national average. The improvements were probably related to both improved surgical techniques and technology and better pre- and post-operative care. However, the study drew attention to one centre, Oxford, which had shown a consistently higher death rate than all the other centres throughout the period under study and, indeed, in 2000, had ceased undertaking surgery for one particular condition, TGV, because of apparently poor outcomes.

The authors of the paper had sent a copy, prior to publication, to the Medical Director at Oxford, who did not dispute their figures. However, after it appeared in the press, a group of doctors from Oxford wrote to the GMC demanding that they investigate Professor Jarman, the only one of the four authors who was medically qualified, for gross professional misconduct by virtue of having placed the information into the public domain. The GMC deliberated for four months before concluding that publishing a well-researched article in a major peer-reviewed scientific journal was entirely proper. Sadly, however, collecting data and putting it in the public domain is one thing, but acting on it is another, and no-one at the Department of Health or, indeed, anywhere else, appeared to take any action over the outcome data for the Oxford cases.

One feature of the paediatric cardiac service at Oxford which bore some similarity to the pre-1995 situation at Bristol was that there was no specialist paediatric cardiac surgeon.

Indeed, all the paediatric cases were operated on by one cardiac surgeon, Mr Stephen Westaby, who also undertook a formidable volume of adult surgery. And as in Bristol, the total number of cases being operated on was significantly less than in larger and more specialised departments. Eventually, in 2009, Oxford decided that if paediatric cardiac surgery was to continue, the number of cases was going to have to increase and, to this end, in late 2009 they appointed a specialist paediatric cardiac surgeon, Mr Caner Salih. Mr Salih was a Glasgow medical school graduate who had trained in surgery in London and then in Australia, where he was appointed to a consultant post at the Royal Children's Hospital (RCH) in Melbourne.

From the outset, Mr Salih expressed concerns about somewhat antiquated equipment, and about what he regarded as poor working practices in theatre. The staff had become used to the rather specific ways of Mr Westaby, the only surgeon whom they had ever worked with on paediatric cases. In Mr Salih's first two months, four babies he operated on had died. He was devastated, as he had never had a post-operative death in his career, and he immediately asked to stop operating and for the hospital to arrange an investigation.

The investigation, which was reported in July 2010, exonerated him from blame. All four cases were very ill babies and there was no evidence of any fault in his surgical technique. Mr Salih moved to a consultant post at Guy's Hospital in London, where he has developed an outstanding reputation for his surgical skill; his operative mortality at 0.1% is among the lowest in the world. Oxford never resumed paediatric cardiac surgery, but one has to wonder whether, if *The BMJ* paper of

2004 had been acted on, or indeed the earlier evidence of poor surgical outcomes, more lives could have been saved.

Looking back on the Kennedy report, its tragedy was that it had the same fate as most of the other inquiries into disasters in the NHS. It was initially greeted with enthusiasm and a belief that it would be the start of a better future, and then quietly forgotten by the politicians and senior managers. As with the Kirkup report into maternity services at Furness General Hospital (see Chapter 2), and the Francis reports into events at Stafford Hospital (see Chapter 9), successive Ministers of Health have seemed to believe that setting up an inquiry is enough. In reality, it should just be the starting point. Few Health Secretaries stay in post for more than a couple of years, so it is rare for them ever to be around when a report that they have commissioned is actually published.

There were two, small, happy postscripts to the events at Bristol. Mr Dhasmana returned to his native India and established a charity hospital for heart patients, and Dr Phil Hammond was asked by the Bristol University Medical School to combine his duties as a stand-up comedian and his column in *Private Eye* with a role as a part-time lecturer in medical communication. But the NHS has consistently failed to tackle the fact that highly specialised procedures such as paediatric cardiac surgery need to be concentrated in a very small number of centres if the best results are to be achieved.

CHAPTER 9

Stafford

In February 2013, the public inquiry chaired by Robert Francis QC into events at Stafford Hospital published its report,[105] which had been ordered by the then Secretary of State for Health and Social Care, Andrew Lansley, in 2010. It was, in fact, the fifth report into events at the hospital since 2009, and this succession of reports into the squalid and degrading care provided to patients meant that 'Stafford' became a byword for NHS care at its most negligent. In 2009, the Healthcare Commission (HCC) had produced the first report into the situation at the hospital, and Sir Ian Kennedy, the then Chairman of the HCC, described it as the most shocking scandal that they had investigated.[106]

Sir Brian Jarman had been Professor of General Practice at Imperial College London, from 1983 to 1998 and, after retiring from than post, continued researching methods for comparing the performance of different hospitals. With his team, he developed a system for comparing the death rates in which he called the Hospital Standardised Mortality Ratio (HSMR). This system allows for factors such as the ages of patients, the

---

105 Report of the Mid Staffordshire NHS Foundation Trust Public Inquiry.

106 Kennedy had chaired the inquiry into Paediatric Cardiac Surgery (see Chapter 8); the HCC was the body charged with the regulation of standards in the NHS. It was abolished in 2009 when the CQC was established.

social mix of the population served and the types of diseases being treated. For example, a hospital serving an area with a large number of elderly people, or one with high levels of social deprivation, might be providing excellent care but still have a higher than average death rate in its patients. A hospital specialising in cancer care might do likewise. The HSMR was calculated by comparing the actual number of deaths in a hospital to the 'expected' number. A hospital where the actual number of deaths corresponded to the predicted would have a score of 100.[107]

From 1997 onwards, Professor Jarman's team published the HSMR for every acute hospital in the country and Stafford never fell below 108. In 2007, Stafford's score was 127, making it the fourth worst performing hospital in the country. By Professor Jarman's calculations, this amounted to somewhere between 400 and 1,200 'excess deaths' at Stafford Hospital over the years.

One might have anticipated that the hospital management would have been concerned, and indeed they were. But rather than question whether there were any improvements that could be made in patient care, they focused, instead, on how the information on which the HSMR is calculated could be improved. On the instruction of senior management, the hospital's Clinical Quality and Effectiveness Group met and decided to take a number of actions, all focused not on

---

107 To anyone who wishes to study this in more detail, I would refer you to a paper by Paul Taylor of the Centre for Health Informatics, University College London, who explains it very clearly and in a way that can be understood by a lay reader. Standardized mortality ratios. *International Journal of Epidemiology* 2013, vol 42:1882–1890.

reviewing or improving clinical quality or effectiveness, but on changing how activity was coded. They instructed coders not to use the codes that seemed to be contributing most to the high mortality score. A review of the case notes for patients who had died was conducted, not to establish if there had been any weaknesses in how they were treated, but to look for possible errors in the coding.

They were clearly successful because, by the following year, the HSMR had fallen to 100, which corresponded to a dramatic increase in the number of patients who had died being recorded as receiving 'palliative care'. Remarkably, the number of patients who died at Stafford receiving palliative care and whose deaths, therefore, would not be considered unexpected, jumped in a single year from zero to 33%.[108] The West Midlands Strategic Health Authority, a body that had ultimate oversight of Stafford Hospital, was also concerned about the apparent number of excess deaths, particularly as a number of other hospitals for which they had responsibility also had unfavourable scores. Again, rather than consider any possibility that things were not being well run at Stafford and elsewhere, they commissioned some research from Birmingham University to see whether they could identify any flaws in how the HSMRs were calculated. One legitimate criticism is that the HSMR only concerns itself with deaths in hospital and does not consider patients who die shortly after discharge.

---

108 A similar system of adjusting of the coding took place at Wolverhampton, as described in Chapter 6 'Shoot the Messenger'. The West Midlands Strategic Health Authority had oversight of both hospitals.

The publicity about possible excess deaths was coming at a rather inconvenient time for Stafford Hospital, because the Mid Staffordshire NHS Trust, the body that ran the hospital, was in the process of applying for 'Foundation' status. Becoming a Foundation Trust created a significant degree of managerial autonomy; it was something that the Department of Health encouraged, not least because if things went wrong, as they are apt to do in the NHS, blame could be diverted away from central government. It also tended to be popular with senior hospital managers, not just because of the extra degree of autonomy but because they could (and usually did) pay themselves significantly more than the national salary scales.

Foundation status had to be granted by the Department of Health, which acted on the advice of yet another regulatory body, Monitor; in 2016, Monitor changed its name to NHS Improvement.[109] As part of the assessment process, hospitals have to demonstrate their financial stability, and also show that they perform well on certain national targets such as waiting times in A&E departments. Once granted, there isn't any mechanism for a trust to lose its status.

In order to bolster the hospital's financial position in the run-up to applying for Foundation status, the Chief Executive, Martin Yeates, had begun in 2006, with the approval of the hospital's board, a programme of cost cutting, mainly focused on nursing staff. His target was to save £10 million from the hospital's budget. Some 160 nursing posts were lost, with retiring nurses not being replaced and £1.3 million being

---

109 When I last looked, NHS Improvement appears to have been abolished; I leave the reader to draw their own conclusions.

spent on redundancy payments. For a relatively small district hospital, this was an enormous reduction in manpower. Additionally, there was a significant change in the ratio of nurses to unqualified healthcare assistants (HCAs), with a much greater reliance on the latter.

Alerted by the data from Professor Jarman's team, the HCC began to take a serious interest in Stafford. They were not persuaded that the apparently high death rate could be explained by 'coding' errors alone and so dispatched a team of investigators, led by Heather Wood, who had a reputation for getting to the bottom of difficult cases.

Meanwhile, a local café owner, Julie Bailey, started asking awkward questions. In the autumn of 2007, her 88-year-old mother had been admitted to hospital for an apparently routine matter. In the end, she spent eight weeks in hospital before she died in November 2007. Her daughter had spent much of her time at her bedside, and had observed first-hand how there was simply too few staff to cope. You did not have to be an expert hospital inspector to see that they were overwhelmed, exhausted and demoralised. Basic nursing care was not being provided. Patients were left unwashed, untended, lying in wet or fouled beds without food, water or pain relief. After talking to customers in her café, Julie Bailey realised that she was not the only one who had seen a family member suffer from neglect on the wards.

She began writing letters to the hospital, local MPs and others. Initially, her concerns were brushed aside or ignored, but she was not the sort of person to be easily deterred. A campaigning group, *Cure the NHS*, was formed locally, and more and more families started coming to her with their stories, all telling a similar tale.

The HCC published a report of its investigation in March 2009. The Chairman of the HCC, Sir Ian Kennedy, described the report as 'a shocking story of appalling standards and chaotic systems for looking after patients'. Sir Bruce Keogh, the Medical Director of the NHS, condemned the Trust's 'complete failure of leadership'. The Department of Health came under pressure to order a public inquiry, but chose instead to order an 'independent inquiry' under distinguished barrister, Robert Francis QC.[110] His report, which heard evidence from over 900 patients and their relatives, was published in February 2010, and recounted a shocking catalogue of failings in the most basic care of patients. 'The standards of hygiene were at times awful, with families forced to remove used bandages and dressings from public areas and clean toilets themselves for fear of catching infections'. He described patients' calls for help to use the toilet being ignored, frequently left in soiled bedding or sitting on commodes for hours.

How could such a shocking situation have arisen in the modern day NHS? Francis found, 'a chronic shortage of staff, particularly nursing staff, was largely responsible for the substandard care'. He noted that morale was low and, 'while many staff did their best in difficult circumstances, others showed a disturbing lack of compassion towards their patients', and added, 'staff who spoke out felt ignored and there is strong evidence that many were deterred from doing so through fear and bullying'.

---

110 He was knighted in the Queen's Birthday Honours in 2014.

He laid much of the blame on the Trust board, their preoccupation with saving money as part of the process of gaining Foundation Trust status and their persistent failure to acknowledge concerns expressed by staff, relatives and patients. But, in addition, he mentioned that 'many people expressed alarm at the apparent failure of external organisations to detect any problems with the trust's performance'. This had not been within the remit of his report, but he recommended a further inquiry to address this. In May 2010, the new Secretary of State for Health and Social Care, Andrew Lansley, invited Francis to lead a full public inquiry to look at why the various regulatory bodies within the health system had failed to identify what had been going on at Stafford. In setting up the second inquiry, Lansley had said to the House of Commons:

'This was a failure of the trust first and foremost, but it was also a national failure of the regulatory and supervisory system, which should have secured the quality and safety of patient care. Why did it have to take a determined group of families to expose those failings and campaign tirelessly for answers? I pay tribute again to the work of Julie Bailey and *Cure the NHS*,[111] rightly supported by Members in this House. Why did the primary care trust and strategic health authority not see what was happening and intervene earlier? How was the trust able to gain foundation status while clinical standards were so poor? Why did the regulatory bodies not act sooner to investigate a trust whose mortality rates had been significantly higher than the average since 2003 and whose record in dealing with

---

111 The campaign group established in Stafford by Julie Bailey and other relatives of patients treated at the hospital. Julie Bailey was subsequently awarded a CBE.

serious complaints was so poor? The public deserve answers.'

Francis began taking evidence in July 2010, with the intention of presenting his report in early 2011. In the event, having questioned nearly 400 witnesses, received 126 written statements and reviewed over one million pages of evidence, the report was finally published in February 2013. It ran to 1,776 pages, made 280 recommendations for the future and had a cost that was estimated at £19.7 million. By now there was yet another Health Minister, Jeremy Hunt, and in his letter to him presenting his report, Francis states:

'Building on the report of the first inquiry, the story it tells is first and foremost of appalling suffering of many patients. This was primarily caused by a serious failure on the part of a provider Trust Board. It did not listen sufficiently to its patients and staff or ensure the correction of deficiencies brought to the Trust's attention. Above all, it failed to tackle an insidious negative culture involving a tolerance of poor standards and a disengagement from managerial and leadership responsibilities. This failure was in part the consequence of allowing a focus on reaching national access targets, achieving financial balance and seeking foundation trust status to be at the cost of delivering acceptable standards of care. The story would be bad enough if it ended there, but it did not. The NHS system includes many checks and balances which should have prevented serious systemic failure of this sort. There were and are a plethora of agencies, scrutiny groups, commissioners, regulators and professional bodies, all of whom might have been expected by patients and the public to detect and do something effective to remedy non-compliance with acceptable standards of care. For years that did not occur, and even after the start of the Healthcare Commission investigation, conducted because of the realisation that there was serious cause for concern, patients were, in my view, left at risk with inadequate intervention until after the completion of that investigation a year later. In short, a system which ought to have picked up and dealt with a deficiency of this scale failed in its primary duty to protect patients and maintain confidence in the healthcare system. The report has identified numerous warning signs which cumulatively, or in some cases singly, could and should have alerted the system to the problems developing at the Trust.'

It is difficult to follow the bewildering rate at which NHS bodies have changed their names. The Commission for Health Improvement (CHI) was established in 1999 and in 2004 transformed itself into the Healthcare Commission (HCC) before it, too, was abolished and replaced by the Care Quality Commission (CQC). It had been the HCC that had finally sounded the alarm over Stafford, but there had been warnings sounded *well before* it took action. As Francis notes, in 2004 the CHI had given the hospital a 'zero star' rating (the worst available) when only a year before it had received three stars (the best), yet no one seemed to have paid this the slightest attention.

Strategic Health Authorities (SHAs) had been established in 2002 following the abolition of Regional Health Authorities and reported directly to the Department of Health. Initially, Stafford Hospital had been part of the Shropshire and Staffordshire SHA, but in 2006 the NHS map was reconfigured so that it came under the newly formed West Midlands SHA.[112] It was the remit of SHAs to have overall oversight of hospital trusts. However, when Stafford Hospital passed to the West Midlands SHA, no-one thought about any sort of 'handover' process, and any concerns that were already on the radar just lapsed.

Francis reported that 'there was a failure to seek out or address patient safety and quality concerns about service provision at the Trust, and there was a failure of the leadership to give sufficient explicit priority to the protection of patients and to ensuring that patient safety and quality standards were being observed there. In common with the system as a whole at the time, the focus was unduly directed at financial and organisational issues and an over reliance on assurances given by others, while losing sight of the central purpose of the service it was seeking to support'. The SHA had told the inquiry that it did not have adequate resources and, worryingly, that Stafford Hospital was not the only hospital in its area with problems, but as Francis points out, 'This again is not an excuse for inaction. Either the SHA had the resources and ability to do the entire job which had been delegated to it, and it failed to carry out that job, or it did not have the resources and ability and failed to alert those responsible to the problem'.

As mentioned earlier, Monitor was the NHS body established in 2004 with a duty to authorise, regulate and monitor foundation trusts and to ensure that they are well

---

112 Strategic Health Authorities were abolished in 2013.

led in terms of quality and finance.[113] Francis pointed out that the fact that the elaborate process of scrutiny, which Monitor is supposed to undertake in the course of an application for foundation trust status, failed to recognise what had been going on at Stafford, calls into question its entire *raison d'être*.

The Francis report made 280 recommendations for the future. As with the Kennedy report at Bristol (see Chapter 8) it might have been preferable if they had been fewer but more specific. Perhaps it was unfair of people to have expected him to have all the answers. That had not, in any case, been the remit of his inquiry and, as he pointed out, the last thing the NHS needed was yet another administrative re-organisation.

Francis, not unreasonably, stated his belief that patient safety must have a cardinal position in the NHS and that staff at all levels must be committed to this. It was a noble objective, and one with which no-one could disagree, but as to how it was to be achieved, he did not explain.

The Minister, Jeremy Hunt, immediately announced two further inquiries; one to be undertaken by Professor Don Berwick, an American with a distinguished record in advocating safety in medicine, and the other by the CMO, Sir Bruce Keogh.

The Berwick report[114] was published in August 2013. It begins with the following:

---

113 Monitor was merged with the NHS Trust Development Authority (NHSTDA) to form NHS Improvement on 1 April 2016.

114 'Improving the Safety of Patients in England: a promise to learn – a commitment to act.'

- Place the quality of patient care, especially patient safety, above all other aims.

- Engage, empower, and hear patients and carers at all times.

- Foster whole-heartedly the growth and development of all staff, including their ability and support to improve the processes in which they work.

- Embrace transparency unequivocally and everywhere, in the service of accountability, trust, and the growth of knowledge.

Reading the report, it is clear that the author is passionate about his subject. It is full of memorable phrases such as 'fear is toxic to safety', but much of it sounds more like an evangelist's sermon or the sales pitch of a timeshare salesman. It is full of inspiring rhetoric, but sadly, and again, short of practical advice as to how to get the NHS out of the quagmire it had found itself in.[115] Nevertheless, an editorial article in *The BMJ* said that 'it should be compulsory reading for all doctors.'

Sir Bruce Keogh, as one might have expected of a man who had previously been a cardiac surgeon, took a different

---

115 I do not wish to seem critical. Of all the masses of reports that I read in the course of researching this book, this was the most inspiring, but it was not the road map which many, including, I suspect, Jeremy Hunt, had been hoping for.

and more robust approach. He identified 14 hospital trusts[116] that, along with Stafford, had had persistently high death rates. He thus arranged urgent inspections, often unannounced and some taking place at night. If anyone had hoped that Stafford had been some sort of 'one-off', an aberration from an otherwise well-run service, he was soon to put them right.

One of the hospitals included in Sir Bruce Keogh's 'hit list' was Tameside General that served an area of Greater Manchester. Conditions at the hospital had first come to public attention in February 2007, when the Coroner for South Manchester, John Pollard,[117] presided over three inquests in a single afternoon, at each of which the relatives of the deceased had complained of the squalid conditions and negligent care provided at the hospital. There were descriptions of patients left lying in their own excrement and of bedsores. Mr Pollard stated that the situation at the hospital was despicable and chaotic. The Chief Executive of the hospital responded by issuing a statement criticizing the Coroner, calling his comments 'unfair', 'unnecessary' and 'insulting' and stating that, 'they may have led to increased distress for bereaved relatives and increased anxiety for patients currently undergoing or awaiting treatment'. Earlier that year, the hospital had been found to have one of the highest rates of Methicillin-resistant *Staphylococcus*

---

116 Basildon and Thurrock in Essex; United Lincolnshire; Blackpool; The Dudley Group, West Midlands; George Eliot, Warwickshire; Northern Lincolnshire and Goole; Tameside, Greater Manchester; Sherwood Forest, Nottinghamshire; Colchester, Essex; Medway, Kent; Burton, Staffordshire; North Cumbria; East Lancashire and Buckinghamshire Healthcare.

117 John Pollard was the Coroner who had first raised the alarm to the police over Dr Harold Shipman, whose surgery was in the area which his Court served, after he had noted an excessive number of Dr Shipman's patients coming to his attention.

aureus (MRSA) infection in the country and an NHS 'hygiene hit squad' had been sent in.

Tameside was one of the 14 hospitals reviewed by Sir Bruce Keogh because of its consistently high 'excess mortality' as measured by Professor Jarman's HSMR score. Over the years, local hospital managers at Tameside had attributed this to what they called the 'Shipman Effect'. Harold Shipman had been a GP in the area and the hospital claimed, without much evidence, that as a consequence, local GPs had become reluctant to allow patients to die at home for fear of being accused as 'Shipmans' and that this accounted for the excess deaths at the hospital. It had been a convenient excuse which allowed them to ignore real problems.

There had been other warning signs too, including high levels of payments in medical negligence claims, outbreaks of *clostridium difficile* infection (*C. diff*) (always a marker of poor hygiene)[118] and reports of A&E patients waiting on trolleys in corridors, sometimes for days on end. Junior hospital doctors had raised concerns about inadequate staffing levels, especially at night and at weekends and about lack of cover from senior doctors. And John Pollard, the local Coroner, had continued to issue 'Rule 43' reports in unprecedented numbers. A Rule 43 report is issued when a coroner believes that matters raised at an inquest give rise to a concern that other preventable deaths will occur in the future and that action needs to be taken. In fact, in the period from 2007 to 2013, he issued more Rule 43 reports, nearly all against Tameside Hospital, than any other coroner in England.

---

118 See Chapter 13 'Hitting the Buffers'.

Prior to the release of the Keogh report on Tameside, the Chief Executive, Christine Green, and the Medical Director resigned, and a new emergency management team was brought in. But the question remains as to why, when it was apparent from at least 2007 that there were serious problems, that none of the various regulatory bodies had taken action?

Another hospital trust which came under the Keogh spotlight was the United Lincolnshire Hospitals NHS Trust (ULH), included because of its high HSMR. The report acknowledged some of the geographical challenges that hospital trusts can face. The Trust serves a population of 700,000 scattered over an area of 2,700 square miles, with poor transport links. Acute services were provided at three centres, Boston, Grantham, and Lincoln, with services also provided at five community hospitals, with the inevitable inefficiencies of services provided on multiple sites. The statistics really hit home: the local population had higher than average levels of unemployment, social deprivation, alcohol and drug use and lower than average life expectancy. The Trust suffered a high staff turnover as it had been difficult to recruit and retain medical and nursing staff, and there had been eleven Chief Executives in 13 years.

In the winter of 2009, the then Chief Executive at Lincoln, Gary Walker, approached the East Midlands Strategic Health Authority (SHA), the body with overall responsibility for the Trust, asking for their assistance. He was concerned that relentless pressure of emergency admissions was making it impossible to meet NHS waiting list targets for non-emergency cases without endangering patient safety. The officials of the SHA advised him that his job was to meet targets. A number of consultant surgeons wrote letters detailing that safety was being put at risk. One, writing two days after the death of an otherwise well patient who was operated on by another surgeon, stated:

'The patient's operation occurred on a day upon which, unusually, three radical procedures were undertaken by the same surgeon on a single extended list. Habitually, one or two procedures would be performed within this session and the additional case was required due to target pressures'. It would have been the standard course of action for patients undergoing this procedure to be nursed in an intensive care unit (ICU) in the immediate post-operative period, but no ICU bed was available and he died of post-operative complications on a general ward.

The letter described 'enormous pressure' exerted by targets, resulting in *ad hoc* arrangements for surgery at short notice, outside surgeons' normal working hours and at weekends, including operations on patients with whom surgeons had had no prior contact. 'This is not only prejudicial to ongoing patient care but presents enormous and unsustainable pressure on the operating surgeon'.

A second consultant surgeon wrote describing pressure to perform a complex, ten-hour operation shortly before he was due to go on holiday and when he would be unable to provide post-operative care. The consultant said that patient safety was of the 'absolute paramount consideration' and added, 'I do not think there would be any defence either in court or in front of the GMC (General Medical Council) if I put the trust's target in this instance above the patient's welfare'.

In February 2010, after a further meeting with the SHA, Gary Walker, who had again insisted that it was impossible to meet waiting list targets for non-urgent cases whilst safely managing emergencies, was sacked, a financial settlement of £500,000 being conditional on him signing a confidentiality agreement.

Following Mr Walker's dismissal, another senior consultant surgeon wrote to the Chairman of the trust, saying, 'I feel I must make you aware of my concerns about the balance between patient safety and targets and inform you that in my view the current bullish and sometimes ruthless pressure from above on the management team in my directorate is unfair and unacceptable. Such a culture that has evolved over the last few months has caused a subtle but significant shift in the balance between achieving targets and the quality and safety of our service to patients.'

Sir Bruce Keogh's investigation was a remarkable feat, conducted like a military operation. The 14 hospital trusts, several of which worked on more than one site, were inspected in four months. Each individual report documented a bewildering range of failings and established an action plan. In one hospital, they had ordered an immediate closure of two operating theatres while they were still on site, pending urgent maintenance work. The constant theme of the various reports was of a willing clinical workforce being let down by disengaged management. Almost invariably there were accounts of managers unwilling to listen to clinical concerns from staff and patients, and of nurses and doctors feeling unable or unwilling to speak up. Eleven of the 14 hospitals were placed in 'special measures', a system where senior NHS managers are sent in to support the existing local management team. In the other three, there was already a new local management team in place.

An additional concern was that, all too often, the hospitals had had a clean bill of health from previous inspections by the HCC or CHC. Part of the problem has been that these inspections assess hospitals by scoring them on a very limited range of criteria, and hospital managers have a tendency to focus more on getting a good score on external inspections than paying attention to what is going on around them. This was certainly the case at Basildon University Hospital, the hospital trust that, of the 14, had had the largest number of excess deaths. Basildon is also an example of how a hospital can continue to repeat mistakes that result in avoidable deaths.

Legionnaires' disease[119] is an airborne bacterial infection which can cause a serious and sometimes fatal pneumonia. It is a particular hazard of large buildings such as hotels and hospitals if care is not taken to properly maintain ventilation systems. An outbreak of Legionnaires' disease at Basildon Hospital in 2002 resulted in a patient dying and, subsequently, the trust had been fined £25,000 following a prosecution by the Health and Safety Executive (HSE). Despite this, the hospital chose to reduce its maintenance budget on the ventilation system, and further outbreaks occurred in 2007 and 2010, with two patients dying and several more becoming seriously ill. The hospital was taken to court again in 2013 and fined a further £100,000 plus costs. The prosecution revealed that there had

---

119 The name derives from a large outbreak at a convention of the American Legion, a veterans' organization in Philadelphia, in 1976. The causative organisms are species of the Legionella bacterium.

been high levels of legionella contamination in the hospital for 15 years.

In January 2020, ten years after his public inquiry into Stafford began, Sir Robert Francis was interviewed in *The Independent*.[120] He expressed his concern and sadness that safety risks in the NHS that he had highlighted had still not been resolved, and that staff remained too frightened to speak out. He once again pointed out that there was still a lack of regulation of hospital managers, something that he had suggested after the Bristol scandal, as had Professor Kennedy.

---

120 https://www.independent.co.uk/news/health/nhs-mid-staffs-inquiry-robert-francis-patient-safety-a9283671.html

CHAPTER 10

On the Merry-go-round

The events at Stafford Hospital are among the most shameful in the history of the NHS. It was a story of poor management, bullying of doctors and nurses, cuts to nursing staff levels to save money and a near obsessive focus by senior managers on meeting government targets. The official reports document abuse and neglect of vulnerable patients on an unprecedented scale. The hospital's A&E department was described as being 'immune to the sound of pain' while the trust's surgery department was labelled 'inadequate, unsafe and at times frankly dangerous'.

What happens to senior managers when things are found to have gone catastrophically wrong? At Stafford, and elsewhere, remarkably little.

As discussed in Chapter 9, Martin Yeates had been the Chief Executive at Stafford Hospital from 2004, and had presided over the cuts to staffing levels on wards in an effort to improve the balance sheet and achieve Foundation Trust status. In March 2009, when faced with the findings of the impending CHC report into the situation at the hospital, Mr Yeates was allowed to leave with a substantial pay-off and his index-linked pension intact.

Mr Yeates did not give evidence to either of the Francis inquiries; rather, his solicitor, Andrew Hodge, advised that his client was too ill to give evidence and that 'he would probably never work again'. He was variously reported as being depressed, suicidal and having Post-traumatic Stress Disorder (PTSD). In October 2011, a statement was read to the inquiry in which Mr Yeates stated, 'My ill health and genuine consideration of taking my own life on a number of occasions has been a consequence, not of the hard work and challenge of a difficult job but the impact of the investigation, the immediate aftermath and the continued harassment'.

Yet a few months earlier he had been well enough to go on a skiing holiday to the French Alps with a group of medical friends. One of those taking part, a senior manager from a neighbouring hospital, Dr Jonathan Odum, was reported as having said, 'I have known Mr Yeates for years and we had an enjoyable trip'.[121]

That same year, Mr Yeates was advertising his availability on a business website offering advice to NHS providers and, in 2012, he was appointed Chief Executive to a mental health charity providing alcohol and drug treatment services to the NHS.[122]

Jan Harry had been the Director of Nursing at Stafford Hospital. She admitted to the first Francis inquiry that she had

---

121 *Daily Telegraph,* 27th November 2011.

122 He resigned early in 2013, just before the publication of the second Francis report.

been present at a meeting of the board when a decision was made to axe 52 nursing posts. She said, 'I was obviously at the meeting but this doesn't stick in my mind'. Mrs Harry also said she had no major concerns about the standard of nursing care provided and that it was not her job to monitor standards on the wards, a claim later described as 'absurd' by Dr Peter Carter, the then General Secretary of the Royal College of Nursing (RCN). The inquiry heard how staff were reluctant to speak out because of Mrs Harry's 'intimidating manner'.

Mrs Harry left Stafford Hospital in 2006, moving to Dudley, near Birmingham, to run a cost-cutting programme at the hospital in preparation for a Foundation Trust status application. After this was achieved, the trust's inspection rating fell from 'good' to 'weak', and the following year failed a basic hygiene inspection. Meanwhile, Mrs Harry had moved to work at a hospital in Salisbury, providing 'management support'.

In 2009, three years after she had left Stafford, the Nursing and Midwifery Council (NMC) finally brought charges against her which included allegations of a failure in her duty of care, failure to maintain a safe level of practice, poor infection control and a lack of governance regarding patient safety and risk management. Mrs Harry chose to retire rather than fight the charges.

Her replacement at Stafford as Director of Nursing was Helen Moss. She began work in December 2006 and was immediately made aware of the problem of staff shortages and its impact on patients, but it took nearly two years before she began addressing the matter. When the CHC report was published in 2009, she was seconded to a role at the SHA on a salary of £100,000 *per annum.* She subsequently left the NHS to work for Ernst & Young[123] as a management consultant, providing advice to hospital trusts facing difficulties.

Of all the stories of managers who worked at Stafford Hospital during this period, the most extraordinary tale relates to the Director of Legal Services, Kate Levy.

John Moore-Robinson was a 20-year-old man who, in 2006, had gone out with a group of friends on mountain bikes on Cannock Chase. John had a heavy fall, complained of acute pain in his chest and was brought to the A&E department at Stafford by ambulance. An inexperienced junior doctor examined him and requested a chest X-ray, which revealed fractured ribs and he was subsequently discharged. He was, however, still experiencing severe pain and his friends described how, when he left A&E, he was also vomiting, disorientated and was unable to stand, so much so that they had had to take him out in a wheelchair. He collapsed and died a few hours later and was found to have had a ruptured spleen, which had resulted in catastrophic internal bleeding.

In advance of an inquest, Kate Levy, in her role as head of the hospital's legal services, asked Dr Ivan Phair, a Consultant in the A&E department, to review the case notes. Dr Phair wrote a report stating that there was no record that the doctor caring for Mr Moore-Robinson had examined his abdomen. He stated that he believed an ultrasound examination of the abdomen should have been performed, and that this would

---

123 Ernst & Young subsequently changed their name to EY.

have identified the ruptured spleen. Dr Phair wrote, 'The premature death of Mr Moore-Robinson in my opinion was an avoidable situation. I feel that an independent expert would criticise the management afforded to him by the staff. There is a high probability that the level of care delivered to Mr Moore-Robinson was negligent'.

Ms Levy did not want the comments to be presented in open court to the coroner and asked Dr Phair to delete the relevant section of his report. She wrote to him thus, 'With a view to avoiding further distress to the family and adverse publicity I wish to avoid stressing possible failures on the part of the trust'. She subsequently wrote, 'I feel such a concluding statement may add to the family's distress and is not one I wish to see quoted in the press'. Dr Phair refused to oblige and Ms Levy decided not to send his report to the coroner, so his opinion was never presented in court. At the inquest in 2007, a narrative verdict was recorded.

The story only came to light in 2010, when a nurse from the A&E department was giving evidence to the Francis inquiry about the dangerously low staffing levels and their impact on patient safety. Ms Levy was immediately suspended and then called to a disciplinary meeting at the hospital in June 2010, where she was dismissed with immediate effect. An appeal against dismissal was rejected in September 2010. Staffordshire police then carried out an investigation into whether there had been any attempt to pervert the course of justice in relation to the inquest and handed a file of evidence to the Crown Prosecution Service (CPS). However, in 2011 the CPS announced that no charges were to be brought.

Mr Moore-Robinson's family lodged complaints with the Solicitors Regulation Authority (SRA) against Ms Levy and her successor as Trust solicitor, Stuart Knowles, who had also been involved in the case. Mr Knowles told the Francis inquiry that, as solicitors, they had an overriding duty to act in the best interests of their client (the Trust) in not disclosing the consultant's report, and that they were not under any obligation to disclose the report to the coroner. The SRA considered the complaint, but decided that there was no case to answer.

This was not Mr Knowles' only involvement in the case. In 2007, when the NHS Litigation Authority, the body that deals with financial claims,[124] suggested that the Moore-Robinson family should be offered £15,000 in compensation, Mr Knowles said that this was too much. The family eventually received £13,000. In January 2008, a letter to the family from the Trust, drafted by Mr Knowles, says, 'I hope the fact matters have been resolved speedily will go some way to enable you to put this matter behind you and move on'. Despite the fact that they had lost their son, the letter bizarrely offered the grieving parents its best wishes for the future.

In 2010, an internal inquiry commissioned by the hospital's new Chief Executive, Antony Sumara, into how things had gone wrong at the Trust, described Knowles as 'callous and unprofessional'. Stuart Knowles left the Trust in 2008 to become an assistant coroner. It would be interesting to know just how he fared dealing with bereaved and distressed relatives. He subsequently moved to work for a firm of solicitors in Birmingham, specialising in assisting NHS trusts and 'difficult'

---

124 The NHS Litigation Authority has now changed its name to NHS Resolution.

inquests and investigations. He died in 2020.

Kate Levy was described as having 'failed to act with integrity, accept responsibility or respect the public, patients and relatives'.

Kate Levy sued Stafford Hospital for unfair dismissal and, in 2013, an employment tribunal improbably awarded her £103,000, a rather larger sum than the £13,000 received by Mr Moore-Robinson's family.

Also, in 2013, the family successfully applied to the High Court, which quashed the verdict of the first inquest and ruled that a new hearing could take place. The second inquest opened in April 2014 and was immediately adjourned by the Coroner, Catherine Mason, explaining that the Trust had failed to provide information that she had requested, telling representatives of the Trust that, 'I want proper and open disclosure of anyone who was involved in April 2006. I will make that clear again'.

The hearing finally took place in September 2014. The Coroner concluded that John Moore-Robinson's death was aggravated by the hospital's failure to provide basic medical attention and amounted to neglect. For his family, coping with his loss must have been made far more difficult by the eight years it had taken for the full facts to emerge. It may have been legal for Stafford Hospital and its lawyers to have attempted to hide the facts, but it is difficult for doctors to reconcile this behaviour with their own professional duty to be honest and open with patients and their relatives.

Alarmingly, and as we have seen many times already, this

case was not unique.[125] In 1999, Carol Tudor, then aged 47, was seen at the Worcestershire Royal Hospital with persistent abdominal symptoms including intermittent rectal bleeding. A radiological investigation suggested a colonic polyp, but a subsequent colonoscopy was negative. Her symptoms persisted but she was repeatedly reassured over the next three years. Eventually, in March 2002, she sought a private second opinion in Birmingham, which identified an advanced metastatic colonic cancer and, two months later, aged 50, she was dead.

Her husband and daughters asked the Worcestershire Royal Hospital for an explanation and the hospital promised them an independent investigation. In December 2002, the Chief Executive wrote to the family stating that the investigation had 'not found any evidence to support your complaint.'

It was only after an anonymous phone call that the family discovered that the independent expert, consultant colorectal surgeon, Jonathan Reynolds from Derbyshire, had in fact concluded in his report that doctors at the hospital had been negligent. He disagreed with Mrs Tudor's consultant 'that her symptoms were intermittent and not progressive.' He continued, 'At every clinic visit during the 1999/2000 period, this woman reported rectal bleeding. He cannot say that the clinical features were not typical of colorectal malignancy because they clearly were.'

Mr Reynolds' report was received by the Trust in August 2002 and, on seeing its unfavourable content, a second,

125 'Hospital accused of cancer cover up.' *The Guardian*, 2nd January 2003.

internal, report was commissioned from Dr Stephen Bridger, a consultant gastroenterologist, who was a colleague of the criticised surgeon. It cleared the hospital's staff of any blame. There is no suggestion in it that he had seen the earlier report, nor that he knew how his report would be presented. The hospital only handed the family a copy of Mr Reynolds' report when threatened with legal action. They subsequently settled the Tudor families' claim for clinical negligence for £300,000, but no-one ever seems to have acknowledged or apologised for the attempted sleight of hand with the reports, and the additional hurt and upset this must have caused a grieving family.

In December 2002, a spokesman for the hospital told a newspaper reporter, 'We feel we have been open and honest in the way we have dealt with his complaint so far.' One can only conclude that some people have different ideas than most of us as to what constitutes 'open and honest.'

Another NHS manager who played a prominent part in events at Stafford was Cynthia Bower. From 2006 to 2008 she was Chief Executive of the West Midlands SHA and, as such, was ultimately responsible for Stafford Hospital. Evidence had begun to emerge of serious clinical failings at the hospital during her time as the SHA, but the abnormally high death rates were simply attributed to a 'statistical quirk.' Little attention was paid to the hospital as long as it balanced the books. As she later admitted, 'Stafford Hospital was not on my radar.'

In January 2009, she took up a new appointment as the first Chief Executive of the CQC, the body that had taken over from the HCC as being responsible for assessing the standards of hospitals, care homes, GP practices and other healthcare facilities. Her salary was reported to be £203,000 per annum.

From the outset, concerns were expressed about her suitability in the light of the emerging story of Stafford, and her lack of action during her involvement at the West Midlands SHA. However, the gravest concerns about her ability soon started appearing from within the CQC itself. One of her first acts as Chief Executive had been to close down the 20-strong central investigations team, which she had inherited from the HCC and which had an established record of rooting out problems. As one former member of the CQC said, 'We were even banned from using the word 'investigation' even though we were the regulator – it was bizarre.'

Things soon began to unravel at the CQC under Cynthia Bower's leadership. The CQC had declined to inspect Winterbourne View (see Chapter 2), a care facility for patients with complex mental health needs, despite pleas from a senior member of staff there. It was only after the situation was exposed on a television programme that action was taken and several members of staff were sent to prison for the most callous neglect of patients under their care. With the spotlight on them it also emerged that, in 2010, they had watered down a report on Morecambe Bay NHS Trust that, in turn, delayed the exposure of the situation in the maternity unit at Furness General Hospital, with dreadful consequences.

Undeterred, Ms Bower took on an additional, paid, part-time role as a non-executive director of 'Skills for Health', an organization that aims to improve staff skills in the health sector. In retrospect, she may have perhaps been better served reflecting on her *own* skills.

When she was finally forced to leave the CQC, her departure was a brutal one. The new Chairman, David Prior, said, 'a fish rots from the head'. An external investigation described her as having led 'a dysfunctional organisation'. There were stories of expense accounts being used to pay for meals at fancy restaurants and for the purchase of prodigious quantities of doughnuts.

Later, in an exclusive interview with *The Independent* newspaper,[126] she angrily denounced those who had spoken against her, proclaiming furiously, 'I am unemployable'. There was no mention of the patients and their families who had been let down by the CQC.

In a final twist, in 2014, with her former deputy at the CQC, Jim Finney, she announced that she had launched a consultancy offering advice on 'reputation management' to NHS and other public sector bodies.

Charlotte Leslie, the Conservative MP for the Bristol North West constituency and member of the Health Select Committee of the House of Commons, commented:

> '*It is a grimly sick joke that two people so intimately involved in running such a fatally failed organisation should be getting rich by advising other health bodies on 'reputation'. This is particularly sick news for those who buried loved ones because the CQC was focused not on*

---

126 *The Independent*, 24th June 2013.

saving their relatives' lives, but burying any bad news.

> 'This is a bitter indictment of the culture of the NHS over previous years, and raises serious questions as to how we can ever clean up the NHS if shameless individuals who were part of the rot are never held to account but keep on returning, making even more money out of the system.'[127]

Another person whose reputation did not come out of the Stafford Hospital scandal unscathed was Sir David Nicholson. Nicholson[128] had been Cynthia Bower's predecessor as Chief Executive of the West Midlands SHA before he left to become Chief Executive of the NHS. As the stories of what had gone on at Stafford emerged in the course of the Francis inquiry, he was widely accused of having paid little attention to anything but the financial situation at the hospital. When called to give evidence, he gave a robust defence of his actions, leading the *Daily Mail* to dub him 'the man with no shame'.[129] Stories also began being published about the lavish scale of his expense claims,[130] at a time of NHS austerity, all the more remarkable as he had been a member of the Communist Party of Great Britain (CPGB) for a number of years.

When Nicholson became the Chief Executive of the NHS, he stated that the last thing required was yet another round of administrative re-organisation. Yet, when MPs on both sides of the House began calling for his resignation, he argued that it

---

127 *Daily Telegraph*, 30th June 2014.
128 He was knighted in 2010.
129 *Daily Mail*, 23rd May 2013.
130 *The Independent*, 2nd April 2012.

would be inappropriate for him to leave whilst the NHS was going through a major re-structure. But with the impending publication of the Francis inquiry, his position became untenable and he announced his resignation.

In April 2018, Sir David Nicholson was appointed Chairman of the Worcestershire Acute Hospitals NHS Trust. It was not greeted with unanimous approval. Julie Bailey, who had led the campaign to expose what was going on at Stafford after the death of her mother, told a local newspaper, 'For him to be appointed to a position of leadership after all the work that has been done to expose failings in the NHS, is a huge disappointment. He was at the top of a rotten culture. He might be good at balancing the books and meeting targets but regarding patient care he's not the man you want as leader. It is a real indictment to think that there is no-one better in the NHS, even after all these years.'[131]

It was not just at Stafford that NHS managers appeared to have been on some sort of merry-go-round. Jackie Smith[132] was the Chief Executive of the NMC from 2011 to 2018. As a reminder, the NMC is the body which has the statutory duty to regulate nurses and midwives. In 2018, she resigned after a highly critical report into the NMC by the Professional Standards Authority for Health and Social Care (PSA). Their investigation arose out of the role of the NMC in the events at the maternity unit at Furness General Hospital described in Chapter 2.

---

131 *Express & Star* (Stafford), 15th May 2018.

132 Not to be confused with Jacqui Smith, former Home Secretary and sometime performer on *Strictly Come Dancing*.

The PSA report states, 'We were particularly horrified that even when Cumbria police directly raised significant issues, the NMC effectively ignored the information for almost two years. Whilst this was going on, serious incidents involving registrants [midwives] under investigation continued, meaning lives were undoubtedly put at risk. Avoidable tragedies continued to happen that could well have been prevented.'

They also slated the NMC for being 'defensive, legalistic and in some cases grossly misleading in their responses to families and others' and for its 'culture of denial and reputational management.'

Remarkably, Jackie Smith was immediately appointed as a non-executive director of the College of Policing, the professional body which sets standards for policing in the UK. The retired police superintendent who had led the Cumbria Police investigation into events at Furness General Hospital wrote a letter complaining that her appointment would be completely inappropriate, but it went ahead nevertheless. She was also appointed to be a non-executive director of the Camden and Islington NHS Foundation Trust.

Not every manager seems able to survive and, occasionally, a manager becomes a useful sacrificial lamb to save their masters from embarrassment. One Sunday morning in January 2001, residents of Bedford woke up to find a ghastly photograph of dead bodies on the front page of their weekly newspaper, *Bedfordshire on Sunday* (BoS). The picture had been taken at Bedford Hospital, and the accompanying story stated, incorrectly, that as the hospital mortuary was full, dead bodies had been 'dumped' in the chapel.

Bedford Hospital is a small district general hospital, which, at that time, was part of the North West Thames Regional Health Authority. Being far from the seat of power, it found itself somewhat neglected and persistently underfunded. For 25 years the hospital had been asking for funds for a new mortuary, but that is not the sort of capital project which wins political plaudits. Every winter, when the mortuary reached capacity, bodies would be stored instead, in an entirely dignified fashion, in the hospital's chapel of rest. However, in order to get a photograph and a story, a disgruntled former employee of the hospital had broken in late at night with a photographer from the newspaper. Bodies had been unwrapped in order to produce a gruesome sight for a picture, but not *one* that adequately represented the true situation.

By the following morning, the photograph had been syndicated to every national newspaper and by 9 am, the Secretary of State for Health, Alan Milburn, was on the phone to the Chief Executive, Ken Williams, demanding his immediate resignation. I am advised that his tone was not polite. The facts of the case, that the photograph was a 'set-up' and that entry to the chapel of rest had been gained unlawfully, were not going to save him, notwithstanding the unanimous backing of the hospital's consultant staff.

Senior officials from the regional health authority arrived on the scene to take charge. Their solution to the lack of capacity in the mortuary was to hire a refrigerated lorry from a local abattoir. So much for patient dignity. Mysteriously, however, funding was approved for the building of a new mortuary.

In 2013, speaking after the Francis report into events at

Stafford, Jeremy Hunt, the Secretary of State for Health and Social Care at the time, told the House of Commons that NHS managers responsible for poor care or guilty of covering it up should be banned from working in hospitals ever again. He also announced that he intended to create a 'blacklisting'[133] system under which failed hospital directors would effectively be 'struck off' and prevented from moving to another job in the NHS. No such scheme has yet materialised, as was noted in 2020 when Sir Robert Francis spoke on the tenth anniversary of his having begun enquiries into Stafford.

Curiously, Mr Hunt exempted Sir David Nicholson from criticism, instead, praising him for reducing NHS waiting lists, despite the fact that it was the chasing of targets which did much to create the 'culture of bullying' and which was so much a feature of Stafford and elsewhere.

---

133 I apologise if the word gives offence. I am merely quoting what he said in Parliament. *Hansard*, 26th March 2013.

CHAPTER 11

Sticking the Tail on the Donkey

While many senior NHS managers seem to have developed a remarkable ability to extricate themselves from disasters and move on unscathed, some of them also seem to have cultivated the skill of deflecting blame onto a convenient junior in no position to defend themselves. The stories of Dr Hadiza Bawa-Garba and Dr Chris Day are two examples of conscientious junior hospital doctors trying to do their best in impossible circumstances and reaping an unjust reward.

Dr Bawa-Garba graduated in medicine from the University of Leicester in 2003. She chose to train in paediatrics, a notorious challenging speciality where patients may become acutely ill very suddenly and where the signs and symptoms of disease may be very subtle. Everyone who had ever worked with her regarded her as a dedicated, hardworking and diligent doctor with an unblemished record.

By 2011, she had reached year six in her speciality training, and had just returned to work in the paediatric department at Leicester Royal Infirmary (LRI) following a period of maternity leave. On her first day back at work, 16th February 2011, she found herself covering the Children's Assessment Unit (CAU) and four wards. She received no handover from the team going off duty, as there was a cardiac arrest in progress when she arrived for her shift. There should have been two more junior doctors working her shift, but staff shortages meant that their shifts were unfilled. Dr Bawa-Garba's consultant, Dr Stephen O'Riordan, was away teaching medical students at Warwick. He apparently had not realised that he was on call. In the middle of the morning, there was a failure of the hospital's IT system which lasted several hours so that laboratory results were unavailable by computer. The only other junior doctor on duty was delegated to spend the morning obtaining results over the telephone so, effectively, Dr Bawa-Garba was covering the whole department single-handed. It was a scenario tailor-made for disaster and, sure enough, it did not take long before a catastrophe arose.

Jack Adcock, a six-year-old with Down's syndrome and a serious congenital heart disorder, and much loved by his family, arrived at the CAU at 10.20 am, having been referred by his GP. He was seen shortly after arrival by Dr Bawa-Garba. She diagnosed him as being dehydrated, secondary to gastroenteritis, and a 'point-of-care' blood test showed that he had a metabolic acidosis. He was treated with intravenous fluids while blood tests and a chest X-ray were organised.

The chest X-ray was performed at noon, but was not examined by a radiologist and was not available to Dr Bawa-Garba until 3 pm. It showed changes suggestive of pneumonia and Jack was started on intravenous antibiotics. The results of the blood samples taken on admission were not available till later in the afternoon and did show some impairment of kidney function, but when Dr Bawa-Garba reviewed him on the ward at 4 pm he appeared significantly improved, sitting up in bed, smiling and having a drink. Repeat blood gas analysis showed a significant improvement from the results on admission.

At 4.30 pm, Dr Bawa-Garba met Dr O'Riordan, the consultant paediatrician, who had re-appeared from Warwick. She discussed the details of the patients whom she had treated during the day. He had written down the details of Jack's results in his notebook but did not ask to go and see him, nor make any further observations about his treatment.

One of the protocols on the paediatric unit was that parents may administer any regular medications which a child would normally be having at home unless the doctor specified otherwise. Jack was a fairly regular patient on the ward, and his mother was aware of the arrangement, so at 7 pm she gave him his regular dose of enalapril, a drug which lowers blood pressure and which he took because of his heart condition. Somehow, no-one on the ward had appreciated that he normally took this, and no-one had told his mother *not* to give it. Unfortunately, enalapril should not have been given in this situation, and shortly afterwards he collapsed with hypovolaemic shock and had a cardiac arrest from which he could not be resuscitated.

There was an internal inquiry at the hospital, but they were entirely satisfied that it was safe for Dr Bawa-Garba to continue working on the paediatric unit, even after December 2014 when she had been arrested and charged with manslaughter.

Four years after Jack's death, on 4th November 2015, after a month-long trial at Nottingham Crown Court, Dr Hadiza Bawa-Garba was found guilty of manslaughter on the grounds of gross negligence. One month later, she was given a two-year suspended prison sentence. Dr Bawa-Garba appealed against the sentence, but in December 2016, her appeal was rejected. One of the nurses, Isabel Amaro, was also found guilty, the court having been told of inadequate record keeping and failure to bring abnormal observations to the attention of the senior medical or nursing team. Another nurse was found not guilty.

The case caused outrage in the medical profession and particularly among junior doctors. There was a widespread belief that Dr Bawa-Garba had been a convenient scapegoat on whom to pin the blame for the shortcomings of the service. Clearly, there had been a systems failure in the paediatric department. There were shortages of doctors, but the consultant in charge on the day had gone away, apparently unaware that he was on duty. The IT system had failed, and yet there were no backup arrangements. How could this be pinned on a junior doctor covering four wards, effectively single-handed?

A further concern is that all doctors in training are required to record in their training log a 'personal reflection' of any clinical incident or near miss that they encounter in their work. These records are intended to be entirely confidential, except when they are discussed by the doctor with their training supervisor. Yet somehow, Dr Bawa-Garba's records were made available to the prosecution. As *The BMJ* wrote, 'How can the NHS ever learn lessons from medical errors if doctors' personal reflections backfire in court?'[134]

In June 2017, the Medical Practitioners Tribunal Service

---

134 *British Medical Journal,* 29th November 2017.

(MPTS) ordered Dr Bawa-Garba to be suspended from the Medical Register for one year. This decision was appealed by the GMC, which had demanded that she should, in fact, be struck off, but a year later this decision was overturned and the one-year suspension was agreed, much to the outrage of the Adcock family. In fact, Dr Bawa-Garba has still not, at the time of writing, returned to medical practice, a sad waste of a caring and competent doctor.

The story was a tragedy for the Adcock family, but nearly a decade on, the GMC has still failed to give any guidance as to how doctors, and especially junior doctors, are to act when they find themselves in a situation where they are asked to work with dangerously deficient resources. Nor have they clarified how junior doctors are to learn when being honest in their reflections that can be used against them in court.

Meanwhile, no action was taken against the absent consultant, Dr O'Riordan,[135] or against the hospital management.

Perhaps, with the benefit of hindsight, one could have suggested that Dr Bawa-Garba should have spoken up when she found herself trying to look after patients on four wards, with no help and no IT. Dr Chris Day, a junior doctor working at night on an ICU in London, *did* speak up. Several years on he is still reaping the consequences...

Dr Day qualified in medicine from Barts and The London School of Medicine and Dentistry in 2009. He chose to train in

---

135 Dr O'Riordan subsequently moved to take up a post in the Republic of Ireland.

Accident and Emergency Medicine, and was always regarded as an excellent junior doctor, consistently performing well above the standard expected of a doctor at his level. As part of his training, he chose to spend one year working on the ICU at the Queen Elizabeth Hospital in Woolwich, south-east London.

Soon after he began working there, in August 2013, he became concerned at the staffing levels at night. He had found himself, with no previous experience of ICU, working as the only doctor on duty responsible for 18 patients receiving intensive care. National guidelines recommend a staffing ratio of no more that eight intensive care beds per doctor.

He discussed the matter with one of the consultants in the department, and then wrote an e-mail to the management at the hospital, copied to Health Education England (HEE), the body that organises and oversees the training of junior doctors. His overriding concern was for patient safety, but especially as he was well aware that there had been manslaughter cases brought against junior doctors who had made mistakes under pressure.

In January 2014, Dr Day once again found himself as the only doctor on a night shift in the ICU after two locum doctors had failed to turn up for their shifts. His concerns were increased by the fact that, in the preceding months, while he had been working in the ICU, there had been two deaths at night which the hospital had formally recorded as Serious Unexpected Incidents (SUI). Neither of the deaths had been specifically attributed to understaffing, and neither occurred when he had been on duty, but they placed his actions into context.

Dr Day decided to phone the duty manager to advise him of the situation. His phone call was witnessed by one of the nurses on the ICU. He was polite and emphasised his concerns for patient safety. He followed it up with an e-mail, thanking the manager for listening to his concerns. Little did he know of the consequences. The manager subsequently discussed the call with his colleagues. Dr Day was clearly, in their eyes, a troublemaker.

In June 2014, Dr Day attended a meeting with HEE for his annual appraisal, the process where all junior doctors are assessed to check that training is progressing satisfactorily. All his reports from the consultants with whom he had been working were totally satisfactory and, indeed, it was stated that he was working at a higher level than would have been expected at his stage in training. Dr Day mentioned, in discussion, the issues of staffing on the ICU.

Three days later he was advised by e-mail that his appraisal had been rated as 'unsatisfactory' and that he had been removed from the training programme. This meant that he would never be able to progress to being a consultant, a devastating blow to a dedicated and capable junior doctor.

Dr Day sought legal advice and took the matter to an employment tribunal in February 2015, which rejected his claim on the grounds that Dr Day, and indeed every junior doctor in the NHS, was not in fact employed by the hospital where they work but by the HEE and, as such, were not entitled to the whistle-blowing protection to which most employees are legally entitled. Curiously, it was around this time that Sir Robert Francis produced a report into whistle-blowing within the NHS in which he pointed out that far too many staff were deterred from raising concerns because of their fears as to the potential consequences.

In August 2015, Dr Day successfully appealed against the decision in the High Court. The judge ruled that the defence in the earlier employment tribunal was not actually valid, and that Dr Day's case should be heard. Over five years later, the matter is still crawling its way through the legal process. The NHS has, to date, spent about £1 million on legal fees, and the questions remain unresolved. Dr Day can work as a locum, but still cannot progress his training. The only beneficiary to date is the legal profession who are able to charge for their time by the hour.

Meanwhile, in 2017, an independent inspection of the ICU at the Queen Elizabeth Hospital, Woolwich, at which Dr Chris Day had been working, reported grave concerns over staffing levels, incident reporting procedures and safety standards.

Junior doctors form the backbone of care in hospitals in the NHS, but they have been left in an impossible dilemma. If they find themselves in a situation where the working conditions are clearly a danger to patients, do they, like Dr Bawa-Garba, soldier on, try to do their best and find themselves charged with manslaughter when things go wrong? Or do they, like Dr Chris Day, raise their concerns and find their careers ruined? Sadly, whichever route they choose, they can be confident they won't be supported by senior managers or politicians.

CHAPTER 12

The Death of the Postmortem

Postmortem (abbreviation p.m. or pm) noun 1 (in full postmortem examination) the dissection and examination of the internal organs of the body after death, in order to determine the cause of death. Also called autopsy. 2 colloq an after-the-event discussion. Adj coming or happening after death.

ETYMOLOGY: 18th century as the phrase post mortem: Latin, meaning 'after death'.[136]

As a medical student at Westminster Hospital in the early 1970s, I would have attended several hundred *post mortem* demonstrations (see Latin meaning above). With my fellow students our routine would be to arrive promptly for 1.30 pm each day at the pathology department and cram into the tiered benches. In the front row there would be a number of senior consultants, invariably including the Professor of Medicine, Malcolm Milne, a man with a brain like an encyclopaedia and a brilliant clinician. If a surgical case were to be shown, Harold Ellis, the Professor of Surgery, would also be present. Two cases would be presented each day, the clinical history being given

---

136 Chambers 21st Century Dictionary (on-line), 2021.

by whichever junior doctor had been caring for the patient and then the autopsy findings were demonstrated and explained by one of the consultant pathologists.

Often, we saw that a patient's disease was of such severity that death had been inevitable. In these cases, we could be reassured that nothing more could have been done. But not infrequently, cases were demonstrated where the cause of death had not been identified in life. This was not because their care had been sub-standard but simply because some diseases are difficult or, indeed, impossible to recognise in life, however diligent or knowledgeable the doctors. An unexpected cause of death was always taken as a valuable learning point, to be stored up for the future. Sometimes a recurring pattern emerged which led to changes in clinical practice. It was at around this time, for example, that we started to recognize the frequency with which pulmonary embolism was a silent killer, especially in patients who had been immobilised in bed for a prolonged time after surgical operations or, as was routine at that time, after a heart attack. The lessons learned saved countless lives. But perhaps of most importance, these postmortem demonstrations taught us humility. We learned that as doctors, however knowledgeable, we couldn't possibly know *every*thing, but that we were fallible and anxious to learn from our mistakes.

It may seem rather gruesome, but those 30 minutes each day were the most valuable part of our curriculum and made an enormous contribution to patient safety. Yet, remarkably, and almost unknown to the general public, hospital postmortem examinations have all but disappeared from medical practice in the UK. I have asked many current medical students and junior doctors if they have observed one and few of them have ever had the opportunity. How could it have happened that a procedure, which is the most essential form of quality control in medical practice, just disappears?

Examining the human body after death is something which has a very long tradition, and which can be traced back to the Ancient Egyptians. After Julius Caesar was assassinated in 44 BC, his personal physician, Antistius, was instructed to examine his body to determine which of the 23 stab wounds had been the fatal blow. This was the first recorded example of an autopsy being performed with the specific purpose of identifying the precise cause of death. In mediaeval times, dissection of the human body became an established part of medical school training as it has remained until recently. As a preclinical medical student at Cambridge, I spent two hours a day, six days a week, on dissection for the first two years of my course, in the Department of Anatomy in Tennis Court Road. Most UK medical schools at the time would have had something similar, but anatomical dissection has also all but disappeared from the medical school curriculum. It is a somewhat alarming prospect that the doctors of the future are no longer being taught how the human body fits together.

It was an 18th century Dutch physician, Herman Boerhaave, Professor of Medicine at Leiden University, who first established the principle of correlating the medical history and the findings on autopsy. He was the first person to describe rupture of the oesophagus after prolonged vomiting, a phenomenon which, at the time, would have been impossible to diagnose whilst the patient was alive. Boerhaave's fame can be evidenced by the fact that a letter sent from China with the address 'The famous

Boerhaave, physician in Europe', actually reached him.

When Napoléon Bonaparte was dying on Saint Helena in 1821, he is reported to have said to his doctor, 'After my death I wish you to do an autopsy ... make a detailed report to my son. Indicate to him what remedies or mode of life he can pursue which will prevent his suffering ... This is very important, for my father died ... with symptoms very much like mine'. His personal physician, François Antommarchi, performed the autopsy, which revealed unmistakable signs of stomach cancer.

In the UK, executed criminals were the usual source of bodies for anatomical dissection in medical schools, but with the decline in judicial execution there developed the ghastly trade in dead bodies, either freshly dug up from graves by the so-called 'resurrectionists'[137] or, in the case of Burke and Hare in Edinburgh, the murder of vagrants and drunks and the delivery of their corpses to the medical school.[138] The Anatomy Act 1832 finally allowed the legal donation of bodies for the legitimate purpose of education and research. This allowed altruistic people to donate their bodies for anatomical dissection, a system which remains in place to this day. The Human Tissue Act 2004 finally superseded the Anatomy Act.

In the early part of the 20th century, Dr Richard Cabot at Massachusetts General Hospital (MGH) in Boston, established the teaching postmortem demonstration, which he called the 'clinico-pathological conference' (CPC) as an integral part of

---

137 Sometimes called body snatchers.

138 In a gruesome finale to the case, Hare testified against Burke, who was hanged and his body dissected in public.

medical education. This practice was widely adopted and was very similar to the presentations that I attended some 70 years later at Westminster Hospital. In 1915, Cabot published a study of some 3,000 autopsies undertaken at the MGH, which was, at the time, and remains to this day, one of the most pre-eminent hospitals in the world. He was able to show that in some 50% of cases, significant diagnoses were identified at autopsy that had not been identified in life. This, of course, was in an era when laboratory and imaging investigations were rudimentary by today's standards. However, over the years, numerous studies from major hospitals in Europe and North America have continued to show discordance between the clinical cause of death and the cause identified by autopsy, of up to 30 to 40%. In about a third of these cases there could have been a significant difference in either the treatment or the outcome.

Of course, a full hospital autopsy involves not merely the dissection of the body and the physical examination of the body but also the taking of samples from the various organs for subsequent microscopic examination and, if appropriate, the taking of samples for toxicological analysis. Finally, a report would be written when all the information is to hand. It is, of necessity, a time-consuming (and hence, potentially costly) process if done properly, but one that, over time, creates a vital repository of information.

Cabot's work helped establish the widespread adoption of the autopsy. In 1951, the American and Canadian Medical Associations (AMA and CMA) established the Joint

Commission on Accreditation of Hospitals (JCAH).[139] This body was created to establish and improve standards of care in hospitals throughout North America, and continues to play an important role in this. At its outset, one of its standards was that hospitals must have an autopsy rate of at least 20%, in other words, at least 20% of patients dying in hospital should have a postmortem examination as a means of identifying and auditing diagnoses that may have been missed in life. The JCAH clearly recognized the importance of the autopsy in quality assurance quite apart from its role in medical education and training, and the continuing professional development of doctors.

In the first half of the 20th century, the hospital autopsy developed a central place in hospital medical practice. Even in the USA, where death had long been a taboo subject,[140] hospital autopsy rates of over 25% were the norm in the late 1960s. As recently as 1979, 42% of deaths in UK hospitals were subject to a hospital autopsy, however, over the subsequent 20 years there was a remarkable decline in the rate of this procedure. Between 1984 and 1998, hospital autopsies in England and Wales fell by 83%. Indeed, by 2005, an article in the prestigious medical journal, *The Lancet*, stated, 'The autopsy has lost much of its authority and now has a marginal role in contemporary medical practice.'[141] A survey of all hospitals in the UK showed that, in 2013, only 0.69% of patients dying in hospital had a hospital autopsy (0.51% in England), and in 23% of hospitals,

---

139 www.jointcommission.org. It is based just outside Chicago, Illinois, in the small town of Oakbrook Terrace which, until 1959 had, rather appropriately, been called Utopia.

140 I recommend reading Jessica Mitford's 1963 classic *The American Way of Death* for a fascinating overview of the topic.

141 MJ Clark. Autopsy. *Lancet* 2005, vol 366:1767.

no patient had a hospital autopsy.[142] In fact, these figures are skewed by a handful of major centres with an active academic department of pathology, which have managed to maintain a significant flow of autopsies.

What was remarkable was that a procedure which had been such a mainstay of medical practice and whose purpose was to act as a form of quality assurance had just vanished, and with virtually no public awareness of the issue, let alone discussion. How could such a thing have happened? There was already an alarming and, largely, ill-understood worldwide decline in the hospital postmortem, but in the UK, the death knell was sounded by events in 2000 and, curiously, the catalyst was the Kennedy inquiry into cardiac surgery in Bristol.

The potential value of postmortem examination is illustrated by an important academic paper from the paediatric pathology department at Bristol, published in 1989, and which was discussed by the Kennedy inquiry. The paper was entitled 'Postmortem audit in a paediatric cardiology unit'[143] and discussed the autopsy findings in 76 babies and children with congenital cardiac disease who had died either under the care of the paediatric cardiologists or following cardiac surgery. The paper showed that, in a significant proportion, there was a clinically important discrepancy between the diagnosis in life and the findings at autopsy. The final paragraph of the discussion section of the paper concludes, 'We attend regular review meetings in which cases are discussed with cardiologists,

---

142 A Turnbull, M Osborn, N Nicholas. Hospital Autopsy: endangered or extinct? *Journal of Clinical Pathology* 2015, vol 68:601.

143 GA Russell, PJ Berry. Postmortem audit in a paediatric cardiology unit. *Journal of Clinical Pathology* 1989, vol 42:912.

surgeons, radiologists, anaesthetists and pathologists. The aim is to formulate strategies for the prevention of the problems shown at necropsy where these problems are avoidable'.

Professor Kennedy's inquiry might have considered whether the surgeons at Bristol were being handicapped by inadequate pre-operative diagnosis or whether this was an inherent difficulty with diagnosis with the technology available at that time. However, he chose to focus on whether parents actually understood what was involved in a postmortem examination, whether they really understood what they were giving their consent to, and the issue of retention of hearts by the pathologists for future research.

Evidence was presented to the Kennedy inquiry from the Chair of the Pathology department at Great Ormond Street Hospital about the vital role of cardiac pathology in the investigation of congenital heart disease, and how the retention of heart tissue for research was routine in the major academic centres. However, in 2000, Kennedy issued an interim report expressing his concerns and asked the CMO to investigate the matter. In fact, the standard consent form for postmortem examinations in England and Wales at that time could hardly have been easier to understand. The wording was as follows:

'*POST MORTEM DECLARATION FORM*

I do not object to a post mortem examination being carried out on the body of...

and I am not aware that he/she had expressed objection

nor that any relative objects.

> *I understand that the examination is carried out (a) to verify the cause of death and to study the effects of treatment, which may involve the retention of tissue for laboratory study, (b) to remove amounts of tissue for the treatment of other patients and for medical education and research.'*

However, evidence was given to the Kennedy inquiry by a relative of a child who had died, in which they had expressed disquiet at the disclosure that hearts had been retained after autopsy, and questions started to be asked elsewhere. Particular focus fell on Alder Hey Children's Hospital in Liverpool. Professor Dick van Velzen, a distinguished pathologist who was regarded as a particular expert on cot death, had worked there from 1988 to 1995. He had been headhunted from a post in the Netherlands to be the first Professor of Paediatric Pathology at Liverpool, with a particular remit to establish a research programme. In 1995, he had been dismissed after it had been discovered that he had removed and retained large numbers of organs from babies and children on whom he had performed autopsies, and that these had been stored in a haphazard fashion, without any evident plan for them to be used in any form of education or research.[144] His dismissal and the reasons for it, however, had initially been kept quiet.

In 1999, the Secretary of State for Health and Social Care established an inquiry chaired by a distinguished barrister,

---

144 By the time this began to come to light, Professor van Velzen had moved to Nova Scotia, Canada. In 2001, he was convicted in Canada of having improperly stored body parts of a child.

Michael Redfern QC, into events in Liverpool, and this was reported in January 2001.[145] The report laid bare the enormity of Professor van Velzen's misdeeds, but emphasized that in their opinion the situation was a unique one. 'We believe that the Liverpool experience is a considerable exaggeration of the national picture'. Nor did the blame fall exclusively on van Velzen. 'Managerial inadequacy indulged Professor van Velzen's aberrant behaviour'. They further emphasized that retention of tissue when properly conducted, is entirely valid. 'Tissue and organs which have been archived are an invaluable asset for medical research'.

The exposure of van Velzen's behaviour, which had been known about by hospital authorities in Liverpool since at least 1994, could not have come at a worse time. The details of his unspeakable conduct, the Harold Shipman case and the Bristol heart scandal were all happening at around the same time, and allowed some parts of the popular press to attempt to whip public opinion into a frenzy of rage against the medical profession. They tried to give the entirely false impression that doctors all over the country were bumping off their patients willy-nilly and then stuffing the entrails into cupboards. The fact is, Shipman and van Velzen were two isolated aberrations, the overwhelming majority of doctors being dedicated and diligent; but that, of course, does not sell newspapers.

The inevitable result of van Velzen's grotesque wrongdoings was the Human Tissue Act 2004, which made major changes to the process of consent for hospital autopsy and for the retention of tissue, either for further examination or for research. In

---

145 The Royal Liverpool Children's Inquiry, 2001.

hospital pathology laboratories all over the country, tissue which had been collected entirely properly under previous regulations, and which in many cases was a valuable resource for important medical research, had to be disposed of. In some cases, decades of research material were lost forever. Meanwhile, the consent process for hospital autopsies was made vastly more complex. A short and unambiguous form, which had been in use for many years, was changed to four sides of densely written A4 paper. In order to be permitted to ask relatives to give their consent, a doctor has to attend an annual training course. Many doctors decided it simply wasn't worth the effort, and trainees in pathology no longer see enough cases to learn the art of postmortem dissection for when they, in turn, become consultant pathologists. Sadly, research studies have shown that the overwhelming majority of parents would have consented to organs being retained for research if consent had been sought at the time.

So, over the course of 30 years, the hospital postmortem had quietly vanished and medicine had lost the most valuable method of assuring quality and safety of care. I suspect that, for most patients and their families, it is something of which they have been quite oblivious. When the bereaved relatives are given a death certificate (officially called the Medical Certificate of Cause of Death), which they require in order to register the death, they not unreasonably believe that it tells the truth; but how, without the hospital autopsy, can they be sure? It will have certainly been written with the very best of intentions but we know that it is not always accurate. And what about senior hospital managers and the various regulators such as the CQC? Shouldn't they at least be concerned? After all, is not safety and quality of care their primary purpose?

In fact, health service managers and regulators have been remarkably silent on the subject. A study from Johns Hopkins Hospital (JHH) in Baltimore has shown that misdiagnosis is both the most common and expensive form of litigation against hospitals.[146] However critical I may have been of some individual managers, I cannot believe that they would really wish to abandon hospital autopsies just to avoid the embarrassment and expense of medical claims. Perhaps, with the relentless changes that have been going on in the NHS, it has just slipped under the radar.

Although the hospital autopsy has all but vanished, postmortem examinations are still performed in cases that are under the jurisdiction of the coroner.[147] When a person dies and the doctors are uncertain as to the cause, if they die shortly after an operation, there is a possibility of violence or, in a number of other specified circumstances (see Figure 3), the case must be notified to the coroner, via the Coroner's Officer, who used, generally, to be a police sergeant with plenty of experience but, obviously, not medically qualified. Now, the coroner's officer is more typically a career civil servant employed by the Ministry of Justice (MoJ). The coroner will then determine whether or not an autopsy is required. If so, a coronial autopsy will then take place in about 40% of cases; in the remainder, the cause of death will be agreed on the history alone. But a coronial autopsy is quite different from a hospital one. Firstly, it will be

---

146 D Newman-Toker, P Pronovost. Diagnostic Errors – The Next Frontier in Patient Safety. *Journal of the American Medical Association* 2009, vol 301:1060.
147 The Procurator Fiscal in Scotland.

the coroner who will give consent and the next of kin have no say in that decision. Furthermore, the family of the deceased has no right to Legal Aid to fund a solicitor to represent them at a coroner's inquest.

A coroner in England and Wales is under the jurisdiction of the MoJ, a notoriously parsimonious body, not the Department of Health, and the pathologist will be under strict instructions to do the minimum required to determine that the cause of death is a natural one. The coroner has little interest in the actual cause of death; his role is merely to exclude an unnatural one. Additional investigations, which the pathologist might ask to do, will not be permitted, often on cost grounds, except in very specific circumstances. To quote a distinguished consultant pathologist, 'The coroner wants *a* diagnosis; the pathologist wants *the* diagnosis.'

I am grateful to one of my recently retired colleagues, a Consultant Pathologist, who is old enough to have performed *both* hospital *and* coronial autopsies, for the following illustrative example. A coroner had ordered an autopsy in the case of a motorcyclist who had died in an accident. It was clear to the pathologist that he had died of catastrophic multiple injuries, but in the course of his examination he noted that there was a significant abnormality of the heart. He requested permission to remove tissue for further study. The heart abnormality that he suspected often has a hereditary basis, and is commonly associated with sudden disturbances of cardiac rhythm. This might have been of the greatest importance to the family, in terms of screening other members and also because it could have been that a sudden arrhythmia might have been the cause of the accident. The coroner, conscious of the cost to his budget, and aware that he had a cause of death, refused permission. In those cases where organs or tissue are removed for further study, this is done with the coroner's permission and, again, the family have no right to refuse consent.

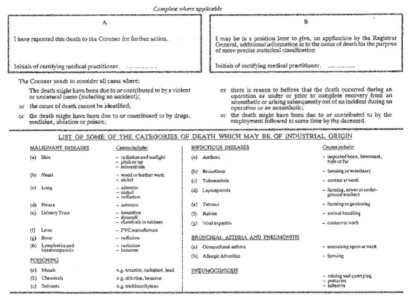

Figure 3. The reverse side of a Medical Certificate of Cause of Death, detailing the circumstances where a case must be reported to the Coroner.

In coronial autopsies following accidents, the coroner may allow blood samples to be sent for testing of alcohol levels, but may refuse to allow testing for drugs, mainly because of the additional expense. In fact, further special investigations, such as histology or toxicology, only take place in 6% of coronial autopsies, and the annual report of the MoJ is quite proud of the fact that, year-on-year, the number of coronial autopsies (and the resultant cost) is declining. Whereas in a hospital autopsy, the pathologist will have access to the case history, this may not always be provided by the coroner's officer in the case of people who have died in the community. A pathology colleague once advised me of a case when all he had been told was that an elderly man was found dead sitting in his armchair. What he had *not* been told was that the house had burned down around him.

Remarkably, for doctors training for a career as a pathologist, learning to perform an autopsy is optional. Of all the extraordinary things that I have discovered whilst researching this book, this was perhaps the most alarming. A contributory factor to pathologists turning their backs on autopsy work is the very small fee payable to the consultant pathologist for conducting a coronial postmortem. The current payment, which has not risen since 2013, is £96.80. For comparison, the veterinary school at the University of Surrey charges £100 plus VAT for performing autopsies on hamsters or budgerigars, and up to £320 for dogs.[148] The pathologist's fee for a coroner's case covers, not merely the time and skill involved in performing the examination, but also for preparing the report, which must be done meticulously, as it may have to withstand interrogation by lawyers in a subsequent inquest. Additionally, the pathologist traditionally gives £10 to the mortuary attendant, he has to pay his secretary for typing the report and he pays tax on what is

---

148 The charge for elephants is £720 plus VAT, provided they weigh less than 2000kg.

left over. Unfortunately, there have been significant concerns raised in cases where pathologists have responded to the poor remuneration by apparently working in haste and making errors.

In the case of Dr Freddy Patel, a consultant pathologist in London, errors in his work nearly led to a miscarriage of justice and, following this and other cases, his name was removed from the Medical Register by the GMC. However, the case that brought his name to public attention was the death of a newspaper vendor, Ian Tomlinson, which shows the difficulties a pathologist performing autopsies may find themselves in. In fact, it may explain why many pathologists are reluctant to perform them at all.

Tomlinson was 47 years old and in indifferent health. He had died having collapsed in the street, and Dr Patel was asked to perform an autopsy. The only information he had been provided with was that Mr Tomlinson had collapsed whilst walking past a group of policemen who were involved in an unrelated matter. Dr Patel identified that Mr Tomlinson had advanced coronary artery disease, and gave a heart attack as the cause of death. He also noted some blood in the abdominal cavity and a bruise on his thigh.

It was just a few days later that evidence began to emerge of the true circumstances of Mr Tomlinson's death. There had been several demonstrations going on in London that day in relation to the G20 summit and thousands of police were on duty. Ian Tomlinson, who had just completed a work shift, and who had no connection with the demonstrators, was trying to make his way home, but had to change direction several times when he found his way blocked. At one point he was bitten on the leg by a police dog, but just continued walking. As he walked past a group of policemen, one of them, PC Simon Harwood, a member of the Tactical Support Group (TSG),[149] hit Mr Tomlinson on the thigh with a violent blow from his baton and pushed him forcefully to the ground. Mr Tomlinson rose, staggered on for a couple of hundred yards, before finally collapsing and dying.

Once this further information came to light, confirmed by photographic evidence and video footage from CCTV cameras, a second autopsy was performed, which identified that the actual cause of death had been rupture of the liver, causing massive intra-abdominal haemorrhage. PC Harwood was charged with manslaughter and, although found not guilty, was dismissed from the police for 'gross misconduct'. It transpired that he had faced multiple disciplinary charges during the course of his police career, mostly relating to excessive violence, and had been dismissed from another constabulary before joining the Metropolitan Police.

The GMC are currently investigating the practice of another pathologist following a complaint from a coroner in the North of England relating to a series of allegedly sub-standard coroner's autopsies. Such cases inevitably add to the grief of bereaved families.

Perhaps most importantly, coronial autopsies restrict themselves to the legal bare bones of the case. They don't allow

---

149 Commonly called 'the Riot Squad'.

doctors and others to learn or for the information to be used for research. For example, in the case of a death following an operation, the surgeon would not be allowed to inspect the surgical wound even if it was suspected that some deficiency of his handiwork had contributed to the death. How are doctors to learn? How are we to avoid repeating our mistakes?

The hospital postmortem served us well for many years as the ultimate form of quality control in medicine. Without the old-fashioned postmortem demonstrations such as used to take place, how are doctors to learn humility and understand their fallibility? In all of this, it is patients and their mourning relatives who are unwittingly suffering the consequences. Families are entitled to know why their loved ones died, and doctors should be allowed to learn how not to repeat their mistakes.

CHAPTER 13

Hitting the Buffers

Dr John Reid[150] served as a minister in several government departments under Tony Blair, before, in 2003, being appointed Secretary of State for Health. It was reported in *Private Eye* magazine that he had greeted the news of his new job with the words, 'Oh f*ck, not health'. Reid subsequently served as Minister of Defence and then Home Secretary, but his reaction was understandable. The Minister of Health is ultimately the person where the buck stops when problems arise in the NHS. They get blamed when things go wrong, and are rarely thanked when things go right, as they do much of the time.

Being the Minister of Health is a challenging position, but it is one that is not made easier by the short time that most of the incumbents have stayed in post. Since the founding of the NHS, there have been 30 ministers.[151] Several were in post for less than a year, and most have lasted less than two. It is all too easy when things have gone seriously wrong, for a minister to announce, often to a fanfare of approval, that there will be a public inquiry. Almost inevitably, however,

---

150 Now Lord Reid of Cardowan. His title of doctor was not a medical one; he received a PhD from the University of Sterling for his thesis on the slave trade in Dahomey in the 19th century.

151 Over the same period there have been 15 Prime Ministers.

by the time the inquiry reports, there will be a new minister in post and the issues which were fresh in the mind when the inquiry was established will have faded from public awareness. As happened with the Francis and Kennedy reports (into the problems at Stafford and Bristol described in earlier chapters), recommendations for future action can be quietly ignored.

Every new minister, when asked for his plans, says, 'The last thing that the NHS needs is more organisational change'. This is followed shortly afterwards by yet another re-organisation, or the creation of yet another supervisory body. The Commission for Health Improvement (CHI) was turned into the Healthcare Commission which, in turn, became the Care Quality Commission (CQC). Monitor became NHS Improvement, and then disappeared completely. The NHS Litigation Authority was re-branded as NHS Resolution. GP Fundholding and primary care trusts (PCTs) came and went. The NHS Trust Development Authority (NHSTDA) was established in 2012 and then suddenly vanished.

Even the title of the government minister has undergone repeated change. It was Minister of Health until 1968, Secretary of State for Health and Social Services until 1988, Secretary of State for Health until 2018 and then Secretary of State for Health and Social Care. Each of these organisational changes was no doubt expensive and disruptive for those involved, but did not, as far as I can establish, help a single patient to receive improved care. What it *did* do, however, was allow ministers to show that they were 'doing something', although they were rarely around long enough to see the fruits of their labours.

It was all very different from the extraordinarily streamlined system established by Bevan when the NHS was created. A management committee ran the hospitals and they, in turn, were under the direction of a number of regional health boards. Essentially, the role of the latter was to organise more specialised services that could not be provided by every hospital. Within hospitals, the managers were administrators, tasked with ensuring that the medical and nursing staff had the resources to do their work. A ward sister, who was always insistent on exemplary standards, ran each ward. A matron toured the hospital on the lookout for any deficiencies. Each consultant surgeon or physician was allocated a ward and a team of junior doctors, called a 'firm'. Patients knew who their consultant and his juniors were, and there was a benign competitiveness between firms to be regarded as 'the best' which helped maintain standards of care.

Consultants had an additional vested interest in being well regarded by their patients in that GPs invariably referred their private patients to the consultants who had developed a reputation for providing good care to their NHS cases.

This may seem to be a nostalgic view of a distant past, but it was certainly how I remember things in my first few years as a consultant. Additionally, we had a consultants' dining room, where we had lunch together, often joined by local GPs. Problems could often be identified and sorted out over a quick sandwich and a cup of coffee. The NHS has not been helped by the fact that now, patients are frequently unsure as to which consultant is responsible for their care, and rarely see the same GP twice. Nor does it help patients that, nowadays, the GPs and hospital consultants scarcely know each other. I remember years ago a patient saying to me at the end of a consultation, 'My GP told me that you don't say very much, but you'll sort me out.' Such a conversation would be increasingly uncommon now.

Not only do patients no longer know the name of their GP or their consultant, they would also struggle to recall the name of their hospital. Guy's Hospital has, after over two centuries, become Guy's and St Thomas' NHS Foundation Trust. The London Hospital is now The Royal London Hospital - Barts Health NHS Trust. Bedford Hospital, where I worked for many years, has suddenly become the Bedfordshire Hospitals NHS Foundation Trust. It must be a boom time for signwriters, and as for the cost of printing new, headed notepaper across the NHS, it does not bear thinking about.

A fundamental change in the NHS, and one from which many of its subsequent problems arose, occurred in 1983, when Margaret Thatcher asked Roy Griffiths,[152] a director of Sainsbury's, to write a report on how the NHS should be run.

Griffiths proposed a much more 'managerial' structure for the NHS. He wrote to Norman Fowler, the minister, stating, 'If Florence Nightingale was carrying her lamp through the corridors of the NHS today, she would almost certainly be looking for the people in charge.' Suddenly, hospital administrators began calling themselves 'Chief Executives', usually with enormously enhanced salaries. They were soon followed by a new breed of manager with a perplexing range

---

152 Later Sir Roy Griffiths. He was knighted in 1985 for services to healthcare.

of job titles such as 'chief operating officer', 'patient experience co-ordinator', 'chief people officer' and so on. Titles often ended with the word 'champion', 'navigator' or 'facilitator', but what they actually *did* was almost always entirely unclear.

In fact, to be fair to Griffiths, this was not his intention. He had visualised a system in which senior doctors took on most of the management roles. What he didn't really appreciate was that the genius of Bevan's original creation was that it was so simple that it ran itself. The last thing that most doctors wanted to involve themselves with was endless management committees.

To make matters worse, the new breed of manager invented an entirely new language, almost incomprehensible to the outsider. Their lexicon was littered with phrases such as 'out of the box', 'in the box', 'fishbone analysis', 'the seven levels of why', 'operationalise' and 'sweating the ocean'. As for what any of it meant, none of us knew and few of us cared.

As a consequence, managers began to spread the fiction that doctors were resistant to change. This was completely untrue. Doctors *like* change and are good at it. The evidence is clear from the dramatic changes that we have seen in medicine and which have readily been embraced. What the medical profession *is* against is pointless and disruptive change. Some managers chose, no doubt through insecurity, and as recounted in earlier chapters, to victimise any doctors who had the temerity to speak out. Griffiths had suggested that NHS managers should have the same sort of professional standards and accountability as doctors and nurses, but that has never happened. Those who failed were able to bounce from one job and one catastrophe, to the next. I know of one manager who had been a failed medical student, and who didn't disguise her disdain for doctors. It didn't make for a harmonious working environment.

The situation created a form of anarchy, where it was often impossible for doctors to engage with managers, and so found themselves unable to effect change when it was self-evidently required. Managers, in turn, all too often found expert medical opinion an inconvenience, which they were happy to ignore.

Inevitably, this chaotic situation would eventually end in tears. In the early 2000s, politicians decided that it would be a good idea to reduce hospital waiting-lists for surgical operations and instructed managers to take action. From now on, patients were not to be on a waiting-list for more than 18 weeks. Contrary to popular opinion, doctors don't like having waiting-lists, but we are all trained to attend to the most urgent cases first, and if that means less serious cases waiting a little longer, so be it. However, that cut no ice with the powers that be.

The process began with the managers asking surgeons to do extra operating lists on Saturdays and Sundays. Surgeons like operating, it is what they do best, but if you do masses of operations at the weekend, then come Monday morning all the beds will be full, and all the cases booked for Monday and Tuesday will have to be cancelled. It had been totally predictable, but unanticipated by the management.

Facing pressure from their political masters to achieve the

required targets for waiting-lists, they began squeezing more beds into wards. The importance of keeping beds well separated had been known since Florence Nightingale had nursed the wounded soldiers in the Crimean War, but the warnings of doctors never deterred the new style NHS manager. Soon, NHS England was being overwhelmed with a particularly nasty form of hospital-acquired infection, *Clostridium difficile (C. diff)*, a highly infectious bacterial infection of the gut, which causes an unpleasant and potentially lethal bowel condition. The management of it involves strict isolation of affected patients, and ensuring that no-one else is admitted to the ward until it has been deep cleaned and the risk of further cross-infection eliminated.

Squeezing more than the safe number of beds into a ward was creating the perfect scenario for the spread of the infection. But shutting wards and leaving beds empty was affecting the ability of managers to achieve their targets. In 2006, there were 50,000 cases of hospital-acquired *C. diff* infection in England, with an estimated 5,000 deaths. The figures for 2005 and 2007 were just a fraction lower, yet, in many hospitals, managers ignored the expert advice of their own infection control teams to shut infected wards.

Curiously, the problem did *not* occur in Wales. This wasn't because the River Severn and Offa's Dyke have some peculiar antimicrobial effect, they don't, but because NHS Wales had not embarked on the ill-judged attempt to artificially reduce waiting-lists, and had not over-crowded wards.

Over 12,000 patients died of hospital-acquired *C. diff*

infection on NHS wards in England during those three years, as a consequence of an obsession with politically convenient targets. A couple of hospital managers in Maidstone and Buckinghamshire were dismissed as sacrificial lambs, but no-one in the Department of Health or at Ministerial level ever accepted responsibility.

The NHS is a wonderful organisation, with extraordinarily dedicated and skilful staff, but it cannot succeed when there is a virtual civil war between the doctors and nurses on one side and the managers and politicians on the other.

Change can happen, as we have all too often seen in earlier chapters in the nuclear and aviation industries. Even more striking is what happened on the railways. The first death in a train accident occurred in 1830 on the very first day of operation of the first railway, the Liverpool to Manchester line, when a train driven by George Stephenson and carrying the then Prime Minister, the Duke of Wellington, ran over and killed one of the passengers, William Huskisson, the MP for Liverpool. For nearly 180 years, our railway system had had a disastrous accident record, but then it made a conscious decision to change. Passenger and employee safety were made paramount, and our railways are now the safest in the world, surpassing countries such as Switzerland and Germany.

Safety *can* be achieved in the NHS. We owe it to our patients, but it cannot be done without an absolute determination to make it happen and transparent honesty from all parties. Whether that happens remains to be seen, but it would be a wonderful legacy to the next generation.

ABOUT THE AUTHOR

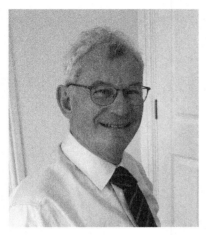

Dr Barry Monk studied medicine at Jesus College, Cambridge and Westminster Medical School, qualifying as a doctor in 1975. After junior hospital posts in London, Cambridge and Bournemouth, he trained in dermatology at the Royal Free and King's College hospitals. He was appointed a consultant dermatologist in 1987 and finally retired from the NHS in January 2020.

He continues to undertake expert medicolegal work in medical negligence cases and private practice in dermatology. In 2008, he served as President of the Section of Dermatology of the Royal Society of Medicine.

Printed in Great Britain
by Amazon

69673632R00129